YOU DON'T MAKE FRIENDS
with Salad

THE SECRET TO LOSING WEIGHT AND FEELING BETTER,
WITH NO KALE IN SIGHT

INCLUDES
HEALTHY
RECIPES AND
AT-HOME
WORKOUTS

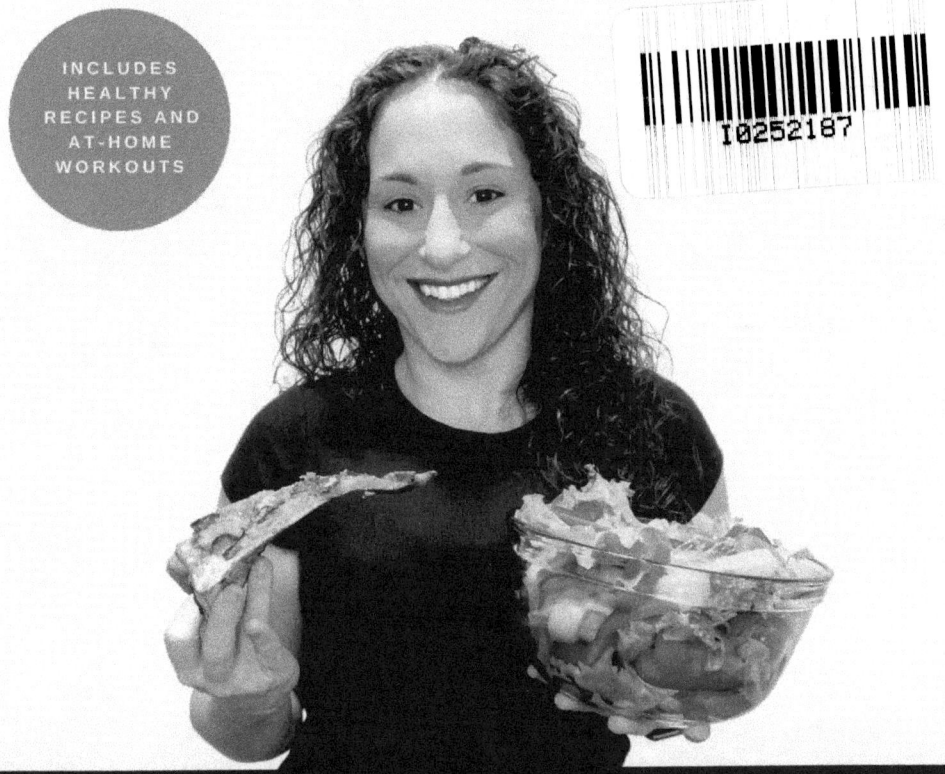

JESSICA GERLOCK

YOU DON'T MAKE FRIENDS
with Salad

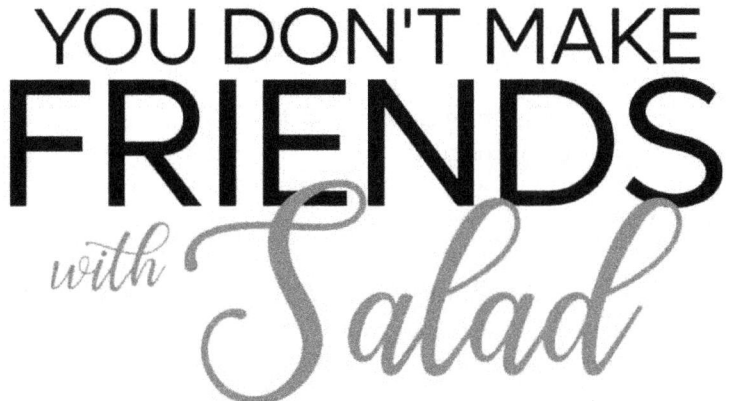

THE SECRET TO LOSING WEIGHT AND FEELING BETTER, WITH NO KALE IN SIGHT

WRITTEN BY:
JESSICA GERLOCK

You Don't Make Friends with Salad
Copyright © 2023 Jessica Gerlock.
All rights reserved.
ISBN: 9781738949106

No part of this publication may be reproduced, distributed or transmitted in any form or by any means, including photocopying, recording, or other electronic or mechanical methods, without the prior written permission of the publisher, except in the case of brief quotations embodied in critical reviews and specific other noncommercial uses permitted by copyright law.

Although the author and publisher have made every effort to ensure that the information in this book was correct at press time, the author and publisher do not assume and, at this moment, disclaim any liability to any party for any loss, damage, or disruption caused by errors or omissions, whether such errors or omissions result from negligence, accident, or any other cause.

Adherence to all applicable laws and regulations, including international, federal, state and local governing professional licensing, business practices, advertising, and all other aspects of doing business in the US, Canada or any other jurisdiction, is the sole responsibility of the reader and consumer.

Neither the author nor the publisher assumes any responsibility or liability whatsoever on behalf of the consumer or reader of this material. Any perceived slight of any individual or organization is purely unintentional.

The resources in this book are provided for informational purposes only. They should not be used to replace the specialized training and professional judgment of a health care or mental health care professional.

Neither the author nor the publisher can be held responsible for using the information provided within this book. Please always consult a trained professional before deciding to treat yourself or others.

For more information, visit www.jessicagerlock.com

I dedicate this book to my family,
who have been my #1 supporters since day one.

11:11

TABLE OF CONTENTS

PART I: THE JOURNEY	**1**
INTRODUCTION	2
ADOPTING A HEALTHY LIFESTYLE	10
PICKY EATING: MY BAD HABIT	17
MY "BEEF" WITH SALAD	27
DO NOT RESTRICT YOURSELF	35
MOVE YOUR BODY	46
DRINK UP AND STAY HYDRATED	56
LEARN TO LOVE YOURSELF	63
SELF CARE: MIND, BODY & SOUL	70
CONCLUSION	77
PART II: HEALTHY RECIPES FOR PICKY EATERS	**84**
Part III: AT-HOME WORKOUTS AND EXERCISE LIBRARY	**103**
MACRONUTRIENT CHEAT SHEET	113
REFERENCES	114
CLIENT TESTIMONIALS	116
ACKNOWLEDGMENTS	118
ABOUT THE AUTHOR	119

PART I: THE JOURNEY

INTRODUCTION

Sometimes in life, it only takes one wrong turn to get you to the right place. If a stranger had approached me when I was 17 years old and told me that when I was 31, I would have lost over 100 pounds and been able to keep it off for almost a decade, I would have been speechless. If that stranger also told that younger version of myself that I would be a nationally certified personal trainer, have my own fitness business, speak publicly to hundreds of people about my weight loss journey, and now, on top of all that, I'd be writing a book on how I did it all, I would have thought you were talking about the wrong person. I did not see this future for myself when I was younger, but I do believe everything happens for a reason.

In elementary and high school, I was not going in a healthy direction, either physically or mentally. At my highest weight, I was 227 pounds and was (and still am) only five feet tall. When I was a young girl, I was "body shamed" by male and female peers at school and camp. This means my weight and body appearance were made fun of and I was bullied. This only got worse as I got older and bigger. Throughout my school years, I was far from a star athlete or even an ultra-smart student. I was very average scholastically and socially and mentally, I was in a very dark place.

I dealt with severe mental health issues throughout my childhood and teen years, including clinical depression and general anxiety. I was admitted to the hospital multiple times in high school for mental health-related problems. It got so bad that in grade 11, I hit rock bottom and even questioned my life. It was a day I will never forget.

I remember it like it was yesterday. I was in grade 11 geography class sitting with my friends, laughing and joking around, when my teacher approached me, scolding me for talking and not doing the work assigned. She said something insignificant to me that I don't remember. The next thing I remember is I stood up with such confidence, like a different person had taken over my body, and told her to f**k off.

The teacher kicked me out of class. That was so unlike me. I was not that kind of student, but I was not myself that day. I was embarrassed and ashamed almost immediately. After getting kicked out of the class, I left the school to run home. I was mortified at what I had done and did not know what else to do. I texted my best friend, saying, "This is the last time you will hear from me. Goodbye."

The next thing I remember, I was sitting in the corner of my childhood bedroom, curled into a ball, extremely emotional, unhappy, and not thinking clearly. Then I remember a quick, forceful knock at my bedroom door, where I barricaded myself in with a large, heavy wood dresser. It was the police and my mom. I remember hearing the cries from my mom on the other side of the door, pleading with me not to do anything and let them in. Later, I found out my friend I had texted told the principal. He then called the police out of concern for my safety.

I will never forget the emotion and sadness in my mom's voice that day on the other side of my childhood bedroom door. "Don't do this. Let us come in. I love you."

I realized, at that moment, that many people still cared about me and I was not ready to give up on my life. Going back and remembering those rough moments in my past proves how far I have come on my journey. I went from being that unhappy, unhealthy teenage girl crying and questioning her own life to, today, being a confident, strong woman who inspires and motivates others to believe in themselves every single day.

From a young age, I never felt like I belonged in most social situations, and I always thought I looked different than my peers. On top of that, like the cherry on top, I was a picky eater from a very young age. As a 90s kid, I took *Homer Simpson* from *The Simpsons* too literally when he started singing the jingle, "You don't win friends with salad, You don't win friends with salad."

Well, I never won or made friends with salad. I have nothing personal against salads, and I know some people love salads and enjoy them regularly, but for me, they were never something I wanted as part of my diet. It took me many years to even eat any vegetables regularly. Now, after all these years and many small healthy lifestyle changes, I regularly enjoy my daily servings of vegetables. It just took me a while.

With age, I did not grow out of the typical toddler pickiness. It was not until I started my fitness and weight loss journey that I started being more open to the variety of food I consumed. From a very young age, I showed selective eating habits regarding the texture and colours of particular foods. My pediatrician was concerned about my weight when he saw a significant jump in my body weight at age two. I was also predisposed to weight issues in my family genetics on both sides of my family. From then on, my weight was something I dealt with, and it did not get easier until almost twenty years later.

Growing up in the 90s, all of my favourite female pop stars like Britney Spears, Christina Aguilera, Jessica Simpson, and Mandy Moore, were thin, beautiful girls who were supposed to be role models for young girls like me. The issue was that I never saw myself in them or any other female pop stars at the time. I now know the importance of representation in the media. Thankfully, the body positivity movement in pop culture is much better nowadays with game-changers like Demi Lovato, Lizzo, Meg The Stallion, and Meghan Trainor. However, there is still much room for growth in the image we display for the young kids who look up to these pop stars, influencers, and famous people.

For the first two decades of my life, I did not know how to love myself or appreciate and respect my body. When you are bullied, and body shamed from such a young age, it is not easy growing up knowing you look different from your peers or the celebrity role models you admire. In some sense, I am so happy that I am not growing up in the current era of social media. It is only getting worse for young girls and boys to see unrealistic/filtered photos and videos of influencers and filtered pictures/videos daily across their social media feeds. These young kids, unfortunately, learn to aspire and look up to images and videos that are not even real, which I find very sad.

When I was in my teens in high school, I was considered morbidly obese or obese II. My BMI (body mass index) was over 40 at my unhealthiest and heaviest point. I had many chronic health problems being considered obese. I had gastric problems, joint pains/injuries, mental health issues, and lived a very unhealthy lifestyle. This was only getting worse with age. Girls and boys got more judgemental, and I was breaking down fast. Something needed to be done, or I hate to say it, but I probably would not have seen my 30th birthday.

The tricky thing about changing your lifestyle and going through a significant healthy weight loss journey is that nobody but you can do the hard work that has to be done to get lasting results. It took a lot of hard work, a journey of ups and downs, learning to love myself, and a roller coaster of emotions. As it turned out...I celebrated my 30th birthday in style in Las Vegas, feeling confident and beautiful, looking forward to what the future holds for me next. My journey was not just about a number going down on a scale. It was about teaching myself to be incredibly independent, strong, and grateful for the life I have worked hard to be here for.

I am thankful to be able to share my story and inspire and motivate others to transform their lives for the better as well. One of the questions I get asked all the time about my weight loss journey is what my turning point was. It took me 22 years to reach my turning point, but the answer was a solo trip to Los Angeles, California, in May 2014. I know it sounds cliché, but it's true. It was exactly what I needed. Looking back, I still don't know precisely what clicked, but the day after I returned, I joined a community centre gym, and the rest is history.

Since I started my weight loss journey in 2014, I have lost over 100 pounds and have been able to keep it off for almost a decade. I did not use quick fixes or go on a highly restrictive diet. I dug deep, dealt with the real issues, and learned to love myself inside and out. This book details how I lost weight by adopting a healthy lifestyle and how you, too, can lose weight and feel great without eating a salad. My main goal in sharing my story is to inspire and motivate others to embrace small healthy changes in their lives so they can live healthier and happier. This book and this journey are not just about losing weight without eating a salad, but what you learn about yourself along the way. So grab a pad of paper and a pen and take notes. Even if it is a motivational quote, write it down, and it may motivate you to make healthier changes in your life.

When you break down any weight loss journey into the simplest terms, weight loss and adopting a healthy lifestyle are not complicated. Technically, simple weight loss comes down to calories in versus calories out. You cannot outrun a bad diet. Adopting a healthy lifestyle is a lifelong journey. Every day you have an opportunity to better yourself and live your best life. It should be manageable and it should not feel like a chore. It is essential to take a big deep breath in, relax, and take small steps forward each day. If you are lucky enough to have a positive mindset and are open to change, you are going in the right direction. If I can do it, so can you.

Stay strong and believe in yourself. You've got this!

******I want to emphasize that I am not a doctor or therapist. Before starting any exercise or weight loss journey, you should consult your doctor first. *****

"BELIEVE IN YOURSELF. EVEN IF YOU DO NOT, PRETEND THAT YOU DO AND, AT SOME POINT, YOU WILL."

VENUS WILLIAMS

1

ADOPTING A HEALTHY LIFESTYLE

Whether you are eighteen or eighty, adapting to and living a healthy lifestyle is helpful when losing weight and improving your overall health and well-being. A healthy lifestyle, the way I perceive it, refers to incorporating into your daily routines regular daily movement, a nutritious and "clean" diet, managing stress levels to the best of your abilities, being socially connected, and getting enough sleep. When I say "clean" diet I mean eating a majority of unprocessed whole foods such as whole grains, lean proteins, fruits/vegetables, and healthy fats, while limiting packaged and processed foods with added sugars and salt.

I also believe to live a healthy lifestyle your diet cannot be too restrictive. The more we are told we can't have something we want it. The trick is to have these foods in moderation and not all the time. Life is too short not to enjoy your favourite pizza or burger occasionally, but you need to learn to control yourself. I will get into the specifics of the "diet" portion later on in the book. Approaching any weight loss journey by slowly incorporating these small healthy changes over time will go a long way, and you will receive more health benefits than just the number on a scale going down.

It is true that the younger you start adopting these small healthy habits into your lifestyles, such as a balanced diet and regular daily exercise, the easier it will be as you get older and health becomes more of a priority in your life. There are so many benefits to living a healthy lifestyle, including preventing chronic diseases, reducing the risk of infections, weight loss, and lengthening your overall lifespan.

One of the more common benefits of adopting a healthy lifestyle is weight loss and maintaining your results over time. The goal of any weight loss journey should never be to be skinny. The most important goal should be to be as healthy, strong, and as happy as possible. It is essential to consider that "healthy" looks different for everybody. Any weight loss journey is very personal between you and only you.

From personal experience, adopting small healthy habits over time has changed my life in many ways, physically and mentally which allowed me to lose over 100 pounds and keep it off for almost a decade. I started my journey by removing sweetened iced tea from my diet and I joined a local gym not knowing what to do, and those little changes have snowballed into making other healthy changes and have created lifelong healthy habits for me. It has not been an easy journey, but it was a journey I needed to go on to discover my inner strength when I was finally ready. You will need help to do the internal work for yourself, so it comes down to a personal commitment to yourself, which is challenging for most people.

A large majority of people who are overweight or obese have some handicaps in their health and weight loss journey. Whether it is an injury, a food allergy, or selective eating habits, most overweight/obese people have something blocking them from achieving their highest potential. My handicap on my weight loss journey was being an adult picky eater and not open to change.

I went to many dieticians and registered nutritionists when I was overweight and they never got me to change my eating habits. Part of the reason was that I was not open to changing them. Also, looking back, it is interesting that some medical professionals never considered my selective eating habits when working on my meal plans or providing general nutrition guidance. Those approaches never worked for me.

Regarding the details of my picky eating habit, the textures and colours of food have always thrown me off. It fascinates people when they find out I have never tried a hamburger or steak in my life. People typically react by looking at me like I am out of my mind or lying. It is the same issue I have always had with salads too. I have tried some salads before, but I was never a fan of them and I would never make one for myself. Salads do not bring joy to my life so I avoid them. It was a challenge, but I had to figure out how to finally adopt a healthy lifestyle and lose significant weight with this picky eating handicap against me.

My weight loss did not happen overnight, but I finally started seeing results and feeling healthier daily. I started my journey by joining a local gym where the average age was 80 so I did not feel intimidated. I started getting more motivated with each workout I completed. After getting into a good workout routine, I started making minor changes to my diet like as I said before, removing sweetened iced tea from my daily diet. I realized there are no quick fixes or magic pills for long-term healthy weight loss. I learned the hard truth. You must move your body, eat clean whole foods, and care for your mental health to benefit from a healthy lifestyle.

It was something no doctor or family member could tell me I had to do. I had to be ready for it. Opening up to making some complex lifestyle changes and getting comfortable with being uncomfortable with my eating habit was a challenge on its own. I had to find a way that worked for me. It is essential to consider that something that works for one person does not necessarily work for someone else. Everybody's weight loss journey is different.

Another critical fact to accept is that not every day will be perfect for the food you eat or the exercise you do, which is perfectly okay. Do not punish yourself or feel guilty when you indulge in some of your favourite foods. Just try to make healthier decisions the next day. Every day is a new opportunity to make better and healthier choices. Punishing yourself, feeling guilty for having a bad meal, or not going to the gym one day will not benefit

> "DO NOT PUNISH YOURSELF OR FEEL GUILTY WHEN YOU INDULGE IN SOME OF YOUR FAVOURITE FOODS"

you in continuing your weight loss journey. The most important part is getting back on track and focusing on consistency. Your overall health and a successful weight loss journey is a marathon, not a sprint. The mindset you have going through your journey is the tone you set for self-improvement and positivity.

Now that I am a certified personal trainer (through the *National Academy of Sports Medicine)*, I inspire and motivate my clients to make those small, impactful changes to their exercise routines as well as their diet, and sleep schedules. I also try to make suggestions on how to manage stress levels but it is often easier said than done. There is always room though for healthy improvements and making positive changes.

There are so many personal trainers worldwide, but what differentiates me from most other trainers is that I have personally been on a significant weight loss journey. I have been an overweight person who wanted to make a change but felt overwhelmed and did not know where to begin. The rest of this book breaks down the journey of adopting a healthy lifestyle in the simplest terms and how I lost over 100 pounds without eating a salad.

It is important to remember that you are the only one who can do the physical and mental hard work to succeed in this very personal journey. It should be approached as a more profound self-journey than just a number going down on a scale. If weight loss is approached correctly, it is a journey of self-discovery, learning to love yourself, self-discipline, and digging down deep to discover your inner strengths. The number going down on the scale is just a cherry on top. A weight loss journey should be about getting healthy, not being skinny.

To quote business magnate Warren Buffett, "Ultimately there's one investment that supersedes all others: Invest in yourself. Nobody can take away what you've go in yourself, and everybody has potential they haven't used yet." A life-changing healthy weight loss journey does not happen overnight. It can take months or years and it only happens if you are ready and open to change and willing to do the hard work it takes. Each day until your last one is a new opportunity to make healthier choices and improve every aspect of your life. So why not start now?

> "IF YOU DO NOT SEE A CLEAR PATH FOR WHAT YOU WANT, SOMETIMES YOU MUST MAKE IT YOURSELF."
>
> **MINDY KALING**

2

PICKY EATING: MY BAD HABIT

Before we dive right into specifically how I lost over 100 pounds and how you can get healthy and lose weight too by adopting a healthy lifestyle, I want to dig deeper into my dietary handicap in my weight loss journey. As I mentioned before, most people trying to lose a significant amount of weight have some handicap blocking them from achieving their true success. Mine was being an adult picky eater.

"Picky eating is typically characterized as eating from a narrow range of foods, rigidity about how preferred foods are prepared or served, and difficulty trying novel foods." (Ellis, 2018) Selective eating habits (picky eating) can start in infancy and continue into adulthood. There are studies which show that if you do not grow out of your picky eating habits by age 4-9, there is a strong correlation between picky eating habits and possible mental health concerns, including general anxiety and clinical depression later in life.

There is quite a broad spectrum of adult picky eaters, where some levels of selective eating on the range are more concerning than others. There are some adult picky eaters that, if too restrictive with their eating habits, should seek medical attention. For most people, though, it is more normal and less concerning not to like certain foods like mushrooms, raisins, bananas, etc. That is more normal and nothing to be too concerned with.

THE PICKY EATING SPECTRUM

According to *Hana Zickgraf*, an assistant professor of psychology who studies eating behaviour at the University of South Alabama, "roughly" 30 percent of people identify as picky eaters. (Shain, 2022) Being a picky eater or someone with some picky eating habits does not necessarily mean you have a severe eating disorder. Picky eating habits are usually classified as part of a spectrum of feeding difficulties that some adults go through.

Picky eating is often a childhood issue that some people never outgrow. There is no single explanation for why some people do not grow out of picky eating with age, but to me, it is like getting rid of any bad habit later in life that needs to be worked on every day to improve. You have to learn to get comfortable with being uncomfortable.

Many adults who are picky eaters are usually embarrassed or ashamed about their picking eating habits, so they are generally very good at hiding their eating habits in social situations. They might even avoid social plans involving food, or they might play with their food to give the perception that they are enjoying it. Many health concerns come with an adult with picky eating habits, including not getting enough essential nutrients, but that comes more with a diagnosed eating disorder. Diagnosed eating disorders such as ARFID can lead to other nutrient deficiencies and health concerns that should be addressed with a medical professional.

THE PICKY EATING SPECTRUM

| Dislike of a Single Food | Dislike of Several Foods / Neophobia | Dislike of Most Foods/ Sensory Aversive | ARFID (Avoidant Restrictive Food Intake Disorder) |

Not concerning and No Nutritional Effect → Eating Disorder such as ARFID (Avoidant Restrictive Food Intake Disorder)

> FOOD NEOPHOBIA IS DEFINED AS A FEAR OF TRYING NEW FOODS. SENSORY FOOD AVERSIVE IS DESCRIBED AS A SENSORY OVERREACTION TO PARTICULAR TYPES OF FOOD AND A HEIGHTENED SENSITIVITY TRIGGERED BY TASTE, TEXTURE, TEMPERATURE OR SMELL.

As shown in the graphic above, some selective eating habits are more concerning than others. Some forms of picky eating habits, if not treated properly, can turn into a more severe eating disorder, such as ARFID (Avoidant Restrictive Food Intake Disorder). It is essential to realize that not everybody needs/wants to enjoy every food in this world, which is okay and normal. Some people have a more sensitive pallet than others, and others are more open to change and trying new foods. All of this is entirely normal and not too concerning.

ARFID
(Avoidant Restrictive Food Intake Disorder)

Avoidant Restrictive Food Intake Disorder is a form of an extreme form of a selective eating disorder. It is a severe chronic eating disorder introduced as a new diagnosis in 2013 in the publication of the "Diagnostic and Statistical Manual, 5th edition (DSM-5). It is not as common as a diagnosis as Anorexia Nervosa or Bulimia Nervosa, but just as concerning.

ARFID is similar to anorexia nervosa. Both disorders have extreme restrictions on the types of food you consume and involve highly decreased portion sizes or cutting out cer-

"THE DIFFERENCE BETWEEN SOMEONE WITH ARFID AND ANOREXIA NERVOSA IS THAT SOMEONE WITH ARFID DOES NOT HAVE THE INTERNAL DRIVE TO BE SKINNY AND DOES NOT FEAR GAINING WEIGHT."

tain food groups altogether. The difference between someone with ARFID and Anorexia Nervosa is that someone with ARFID does not have the internal drive to be skinny and does not fear gaining weight. ARFID involves a more negative relationship with the foods you consume rather than having a negative relationship with yourself. Since there are some similarities, ARFID often gets misdiagnosed.

If you are willing and open to changing your eating habits slowly, making minor changes is usually the best way to handle most picky eaters. Still, it is a process that only happens after a period of time. Again, you have to be open to new foods and healthy changes. If you are a picky eater, then you should focus on improving daily by introducing one small healthy change one at a time without overwhelming yourself. If you get too overwhelmed, you will give up and won't be as willing to make changes in the future and try new foods, so go slow. Keep in mind that slow and steady wins the race.

For some people, including myself, colour is a common deterrent that can cause people to avoid consuming certain foods. There is a common "diet" that picky eaters seem to lean towards due to the lack of colour in their foods. This is called the Beige Diet.

THE BEIGE DIET

The beige diet is described as a diet high in refined carbohydrates, lacking colour, and low in fruits and vegetables. This colour-lacking diet usually includes refined carbohydrates, such as potatoes, pasta, rice, and white bread. It is a highly caloric non-balanced diet that does not have many nutrients which a whole food balanced diet includes. This colour-lacking diet is not suitable for your long-term health.

Many people worldwide are considered visual learners. One of the most significant deterrents for many picky eaters is the visual appearance and colour of the food they consume. When first introduced to food, it is common for your first sense to activate and internally judge the food with sight. It is like a first date. It would be best if you liked what you see at first glance to go further. If you like the way the food looks, there is a higher chance you will consume it.

One of my picky eating issues is the idea of eating red meat due to its colour and texture. Since I am a very visual person, the look of red meat, cooked or raw is very unappealing to me. The thought of actually eating a piece of brown meat that is bleeding is far from appetizing. I also have an issue with the texture of meat, especially chopped meat, as in a chicken burger, although I have tried them. As hard as it is for most to believe, I have never eaten a hamburger or steak. I do eat other coloured foods such as salmon, green beans, berries, broccoli, apples, oranges, watermelon, bananas, etc.,

The beige diet can be concerning as it can cause serious nutrient deficits. It is important to consume a balanced diet and include all the macronutrient groups such as your proteins, fats, and healthy carbohydrates to receive all the health benefits of a whole food diet.

MENTAL ILLNESS AND PICKY EATING

There have been studies that show a correlation between mental health disorders, including autism, OCD (Obsessive Compulsive Disorder), ADHD, and picky eating. For example: "An estimated 46% - 89% of children with Autism Spectrum Disorder have feeding problems" (Bandini, 2017). This includes selective eating habits such as extreme picky eating. Extreme cases of picky eating habits or feeding difficulties from a young age can also be a sign of other mental health issues later on in life.

There also have been studies that show a connection between someone with general anxiety or clinical depression and selective eating habits. A 2004 study by the *Anxiety and Depression Association of America* found that 2/3 of people with eating disorders suffer from an anxiety disorder at some point in their lives. Stress and anxiety are commonly known to suppress a person's appetite or cause them to make poor food choices and binge eat. There are some treatments available that are recommended for those dealing with extremely picky eating due to mental health illnesses, including exposure therapy, CBT (Cognitive Behaviour Therapy), or just having a consultation and working with your local registered dieticians and nutritionists to find a solution that works for you.

If your picky eating habits affect your life negatively or your physical or mental health is impacted by your fear of changing your eating habits, then it would be a good idea to contact your doctor or a health care professional as soon as possible. If it helps you be your best self, conquer your fear of trying new things, and possibly even enjoy them.

HELPFUL TIPS FOR PICKY EATERS

1. Introduce one new food at a time. Refrain from overwhelming yourself with introducing a plate full of new foods, which will only discourage you.
2. Try pairing new foods you introduce to your diet with familiar foods you know you like.
3. Incorporate regular exposure to new foods. You will be more successful if no one pressures you and you are open to trying something new.
4. Prepare foods differently if you do not like a particular food prepared a certain way. For example, if you do not like cooked vegetables, try them raw or blended in a soup or smoothie.
5. When introducing new foods, be in a comfortable environment, such as your home or a friend's house, where you are relaxed and around people who will support you and not judge you.
6. Do not give up after trying food once.
7. Commit to eating only a few bites when introducing a new food.
8. Try new recipes and have fun with them. Cooking and trying new foods should be a positive experience.

9. Do not overthink trying a new food too much. What is the worst that is going to happen?
10. Have a positive mindset, be open to change and keep moving forward!

"GREAT PEOPLE DO THINGS BEFORE THEY'RE READY. THEY DO THINGS BEFORE THEY KNOW THEY CAN DO IT. DOING WHAT YOU'RE AFRAID OF, GETTING OUT OF YOUR COMFORT ZONE, TAKING RISKS LIKE THAT-
THAT'S WHAT LIFE IS."

AMY POEHLER

3

MY "BEEF" WITH SALAD

Before I share my issue or personal "beef" with salads, I want to clarify that this is nothing personal against anybody who enjoys salad. Salads were just never for me and never brought enjoyment into my life. Even though I did not regularly eat salads on my weight loss journey, the common notion is that you must eat lots and lots of salads to lose weight and get healthy. Well, I broke that rule.

I have always been the girl who does not follow rules and enjoys doing things my way. Since I was a little girl, I was never a fan of salads. Yes, I have tried a salad before. Still, besides a Caesar Salad, which technically could be considered one of the most unhealthy and non-nutrient-containing salads there are, I am not a fan of salads. I am proud to say I did not eat them regularly to lose weight or to keep off the weight long-term.

Before starting my weight loss journey, I had zero interest in eating salads or any vegetables. The odd time, as I mentioned above, I would order a Caesar salad, usually at a restaurant, possibly thinking I was making a healthier choice. I now know I was not. Growing up as an overweight girl, I saw many health professionals who tried to figure out my weight problems. Still, it was only when I was ready to make a significant change that I started to get comfortable being uncomfortable and began incorporating vegetables into my diet.

Over the years of being overweight, many registered nutritionists and dieticians tried to get me to eat all these salads and vegetables as part of the meal plans they would create for me. I was not interested at all. I knew in my head that these meal plans would not work before I even left their office. All their knowledge and technical information went in one ear and out the other.

For many years I was in my comfort zone with my eating and not ready to get uncomfortable, especially with the food I ate. I saw more than a handful of registered dieticians and nutritionists during those challenging years and none of them got me hooked on making a change. It took many years, but in the end, it had to be me who was ready to change my habits.

Even now, I prefer raw vegetables to cooked ones due to the texture, but that is okay as long as I get my daily servings of vegetables. If you are like me and are picky with the textures of the food, you can prepare your vegetables in many different ways to at least get 4-5 servings of vegetables a day. You can eat them raw, cook them, put them in smoothies, put them in soups, juice some of them, and figure out what you prefer and how you will incorporate your daily servings of vegetables into your meal plans without having to eat a salad. The key is to get creative and have fun with it.

SALADS ARE NOT ALWAYS HEALTHY

Personally, being a picky eater, one of the reasons I am not interested in eating salads is because of the mixture of different food groups, textures, and colours in them. Some salads can actually be considered very unhealthy in many ways. Now, when I think about it, I think the reason I was willing to eat Caesar salads was because of it being pretty simple...in general it was lettuce, dressing and croutons. The main thing it didn't have was any extra vegetables. Did you know there are some salads from large restaurant chains that are more calories than a *McDonald's* Big Mac?

For example, the Taco Salad from *Wendy's* is 670 calories with 1970 mg of sodium, 61 g of carbohydrates and 36 g of fat. *Wendy's* Taco Salad is almost 100 calories more than the 570-calorie Big Mac and more than double the amount of sodium. Another example is the appetizer Caesar Salad at the *Cheesecake Factory* which clocks in at 860 calories, and if you add Chicken, it jumps to 1090 calories. That is almost the same amount of calories as two big macs.

Due to diet culture, people seem to think that every salad is a healthier choice than their favourite comfort foods, but the truth is that they aren't always. Being able to look out for signs that a salad is not as healthy for you as you may think is looking for ingredients added such as processed meats like deli meat or bacon, added croutons or wontons, creamy or heavily oily dressings, and fried meats. Also sometimes salads have more than one of these ingredients in them.

Dressings are usually the big killer of a healthy salad. Store-bought, regular-fat salad dressings often turn a salad from healthy to unhealthy really fast. Regular fat salad dressings can be high in calories, sodium, added sugar, saturated fat, and added preservatives. Usually, the healthier salad dressings are vinaigrette-based, such as balsamic or oil and vinegar. In contrast, creamy dressings such as Caesar, Ranch, and Thousand Island usually are highly caloric and unhealthier for you.

Do yourself a favour and do some research the next time you eat your favourite salad. Find out what is in the salad, if it has all your macronutrients, how much fat and sodium are in it, and how many calories it has. Use an internal checklist to ensure the salad is

MACRONUTRIENTS - DEFINED AS NUTRIENTS THAT YOUR BODY USES IN THE LARGEST AMOUNTS. ALSO NUTRIENTS THAT YOUR BODY GETS ITS ENERGY FROM.

a balanced healthy meal with all your macronutrients included.

BALANCE YOUR SALADS

Any balanced meal, including salads for those who enjoy salads, should include proper portion sizes of lean protein, healthy fat and healthy carbohydrates, which can consist of fresh fruits and vegetables. Ensure that the important part of a salad should be a portion size of a clean protein source. Sorry, but fried chicken does not count.

Adding the proper portion sizes of protein (animal or plant-based, whichever you prefer), which is the size of a deck of cards, should be the most important ingredient you include. Healthy protein sources you can add to a salad include grilled chicken, grilled steak, tuna, seafood, salmon, tofu, etc. A proper portion size of healthy fat (which includes salad dressing) for your salad should be the size of your thumbprint. It is good to know one gram of fat has nine calories, double what a protein or carbohydrate has. Regarding vegetables, you can add two whole handfuls, and you do not have to be so strict with portion sizes regarding non-starchy vegetables.

The common notion is that most people think that because most salads contain lettuce, which is a vegetable, all salads are healthy. In regards to lettuce, it is good to keep in mind that the darker green the lettuce is the more nutrients it contains. For example, iceberg lettuce does not contain that many nutrients compared to darker green lettuce such as romaine. The problem is that when you take the lettuce and add fried chicken or processed bacon, creamy dressings, or fried croutons and wontons, it makes the nutrient-lacking lettuce even more unhealthy. Another problem is that you are never delighted at the end of the meal, and you will usually want something else to satisfy your hunger. That could, unfortunately, assist in making other bad food choices in what else you decide to consume.

HOW TO MAKE SURE YOUR SALAD IS HEALTHY

If you are someone who likes salads or has ever craved a salad and you have a weight loss goal, there are ways to ensure your salad is satisfying and healthy, filled with lean protein, healthy fats, and good complex carbohydrates. As shown in the chart below, there are easy switch-outs to make your salad a healthier choice and a more satisfying meal. If you have a weight loss goal or want to make healthier choices, avoid adding to your salad: processed meats, including deli meat and bacon, as well as avoid fried croutons or fried wontons and instead add a "crunch" factor by adding some nuts, seeds, or rice noodles.

As you can already tell by the title of this book, I am not a fan of salads, and I am not ashamed of that. Most salads could be more visually appealing, and to me, a salad is just a mix of different food groups in a bowl covered in dressing. Being a visual eater, I need help with the idea of a salad. I do not judge people who love salads, but it is essential to ensure that your salad is balanced, including healthy fats, protein, and carbohydrates, if you have a weight loss goal. Otherwise, your salad could be as many calories as a Big Mac or Whopper combo but less enjoyable and less satisfying.

HEALTHIER SALAD SWITCH-OUTS

Unhealthy Ingredients	Healthier Ingredients
Fried Chicken or Fried Fish	Grilled or broiled chicken or fish
High Fat Dressings such as Ranch, French, etc.	Low-fat dressing or olive oil, lemon/lime juice, balsamic vinegar
Bacon	Oven roasted nuts or seeds
Croutons/Wontons/Chow Mein Fried Noodles	Nuts or Seeds including walnuts or almonds or sunflower/chia seeds
Whole Fat Cheese	Low-fat cheese with other proteins
Dried Fruit	Fresh fruit
Iceberg or other pale lettuce	Darker lettuce (romaine) or Leafy Greens (spring mix/baby spinach/arugula)
White Potatoes	Sweet potatoes
Canned Goods	Good in moderation as often are high in sodium

"A SALAD IS NOT A MEAL; IT IS A STYLE."

FRAN LEBOWITZ

4

DO NOT RESTRICT YOURSELF

According to the World Health Organization (WHO), a healthy lifestyle is defined as, "A way of living that lowers the risk of being seriously ill or dying early" (World Health Organization, 1999). The rest of the book will go in-depth on the steps to adopting a healthy lifestyle and show you the overall journey of my one-hundred-pound weight loss. Even sitting here writing this book, I cannot believe my accomplishment of losing over 100 pounds and keeping it off for almost a decade. As a certified personal trainer who does this for a living, it is rarer than most people realize. Statistics show that nearly 90% of people quit in the first three months of starting a new fitness and/or weight loss journey.

It is known that some people do not like making complex life changes. Some people find it even harder to resist external temptations. In any transformative weight loss journey, it is all about getting used to change, learning about willpower, getting out of your comfort zone, and accepting a lot of delicious temptations that you sometimes need to know to say no to. This journey comes down to you versus you.

> "EVERYONE IN THIS WORLD IS DIFFERENT, WHICH IS BEAUTIFUL, AND EVERYONE'S JOURNEY IN TACKLING THEIR HEALTH AND FITNESS GOALS WILL BE DIFFERENT."

Everyone in this world is different, which is beautiful, and everyone's journey in tackling their health and fitness goals will be different. I always say that if there is a will, there is a way. Depending on your lifestyle, job, family life, and schedule, you must find a way to succeed in your journey that works just for you.

There are a million ways to lose weight in unhealthy ways and tons of quick fixes that might help you temporarily lose weight. From a personal and professional point of view, to lose weight healthily and keep it off for an extended period, there is only one way, an actual healthy lifestyle change. It does not happen overnight; however, it will help you succeed overall in your weight loss journey.

If any health care professional right now, including doctors, dieticians, or nutritionists, told me not to eat my favourite food, like Chinese food, chicken fingers and fries or have some pizza occasionally, I would have fired them right away. I am one of those people who, if you tell me "no," I only want it more. In a weight loss journey, you should never restrict yourself from your favourites for extended periods because that is not manageable or enjoyable for the rest of your life. Eventually, you will fold and binge more than you would have by satisfying the original craving.

> **PLAN AHEAD**
> When you plan your meals in advance, it is more likely you'll make better quality choices and eat proper portions.

Since I started my journey, I have changed my mindset to the idea that you do not have to restrict yourself to anything you enjoy, but you need to change how you think so that it is not all or nothing and everything is in moderation. When you first begin your weight loss journey, it is helpful to be more disciplined regarding your eating habits, which is essential to get into a healthy routine. After some time, you can start slowly reintroducing some of your favourite foods and indulge occasionally. Make sure you start slow and take small baby steps forward because, in the end, there is no deadline to living a healthy lifestyle.

It is also a helpful tip to not compare your journey to anybody else's. Start your healthy lifestyle by choosing only one area where you want to start your journey. Whether it is a small healthy change, such as trading in sugar drinks like soda/pop for sparking water or flat water or beginning to incorporate some form of regular daily exercise. Start with one area. These small, manageable lifestyle changes will substantially impact your overall success on your weight loss journey and overall health. Your age does not matter. Everybody has a new and beautiful opportunity to better themselves and live a healthier, happier life every single day.

I remember what my first healthy lifestyle change was. The small achievable goal was to drop sweetened iced tea from my diet and replace it with drinking water. That was all I had to do. The first step of action was to stop buying it and have it in my house. I used the mentality of out of sight, out of mind, and I never even missed it.

I never restricted myself completely. I would continue to go out to a restaurant and order an iced tea as a treat, but eventually, the urge and the sweet tooth disappeared. Those empty calories that I was consuming turned into sugar and, in the end, added to an increase in my body weight.

That small change started my healthy lifestyle. Getting rid of drinking empty calories, combined with all my other small lifestyle changes, added to a balanced healthy lifestyle that has lasted almost a decade. I still, occasionally, have a sweetened iced tea as a special treat if I am out at a restaurant, but I never crave it anymore or "need" it as I once did.

EVERYTHING IN MODERATION

Almost every aspect of your life, including what you eat and how much you exercise, should all be in moderation and balance.

When it comes to your diet, if you want a couple of slices of pizza occasionally, that is totally okay. You should enjoy every last bite, and if you want chocolate cake another day, you should go for it, but it is important to keep in mind that if your goal is any weight loss, it comes down to calories consumed versus calories burned, so it is important to space out your "cheat" meals.

Some fitness trainers will say weight loss is 80/20, which means that 80% of weight loss comes from your diet and 20% comes from exercise. After going through my weight loss transformation, my theory is that weight loss is about giving 100% to your diet, 100% to your workouts, and 100% to a positive mindset. You must put 100% into all three areas for major long-term success. You also have to be open to change and be willing to give yourself up to the lifestyle because that is when growth, success, and actual long-term results will happen.

PORTION CONTROL

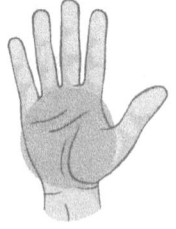
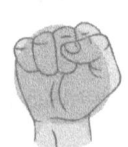
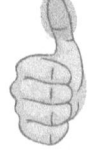
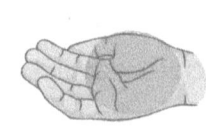

Protein	Grains/Starchy Carbohydrates/ Fruits	Fat	Vegetables
A portion size of protein is the size of the palm of your hand.	Limit portion to the size of your fist for grains, starches, or fruit.	Limit fat to an amount the size of your thumbprint.	Choose as much as you can hold in both hands. Brightly coloured vegetables are always preferred.

Another critical concept to incorporate into your healthy lifestyle for a balanced diet is portion control. Portion control is the basic idea that instead of eating a whole cake, only have one slice. Reading food labels is a great way to be more aware and see the proper portion sizes on packaged foods.

Regarding proper portion sizes, every macronutrient has a different portion size. (Refer to the Macronutrient cheat sheet in the back of the book.) When it comes to protein, a single piece is the size of a deck of cards or the palm of your hand. When it comes to healthy fats, proper portion size is the size of an average thumbprint. An effective strategy for being mindful of portion sizes if your goal is weight loss is to increase the proportion of low-calorie foods in your diet while limiting portions of high-calorie foods. If you lower your daily caloric intake, you can eat satisfying portions while managing your body weight (Rolls BJ, 2014).

It is helpful to be mindful of the quality of calories you consume and not partake in mindless eating. Making these small, impactful changes and being aware of what you are eating will significantly impact your weight loss journey. For some people, the idea of any change can be extremely terrifying, so most stay in their comfort zone and never change. You need to start getting comfortable with being uncomfortable if you want to see real change. Being open to change is essential to prevent you from becoming overwhelmed with all these lifestyle changes. Real change happens outside of your comfort zone.

Another helpful tip is to go into your weight loss journey, with the idea that the key to long-term weight loss is making small healthy, impactful changes and consistency over time. Also, accept that finding the right custom recipe for your long-term weight loss success takes time and a lot of trial and error. It is essential to enjoy the journey and appreciate what you learn along the way. It is helpful to use some form to track your progress, whether it is before and after photos, body measurements, the number on the scale, or whatever you are most comfortable with to track your progress. Everybody's journey will be different, and not one single way will work for everyone, but figuring out what works for you, controlling your calories in versus calories out and participating in a form of exercise you enjoy is a massive factor in the success of your weight loss goals.

As a personal trainer, when I get a new client just starting any fitness journey, I suggest in the initial consultation that we begin this journey by making a SMART goal.

SMART GOALS

A smart goal is described as a Specific, Measurable, Attainable, Realistic, and Timely goal. With anyone just starting a weight loss and fitness journey, this is the best place to start. Evidence suggests that developing a SMART goal before a weight loss journey can be highly effective in weight management and nutrition programs. (Pearson, 2012) It is essential to be realistic and honest with what you are willing to do to achieve those goals. You are not going to make significant changes if you are not going to do the hard work for it. For example, you will not lose fifty pounds in two months by not changing your diet and only incorporating a light and low-impact workout once a week for less than thirty minutes. That is not a realistic goal.

Once you have set your SMART goal and figured out what actions and changes you will need to accomplish to achieve those goals, you are ready to go. This is when your actions mean more than just words. Whatever that first step for you is, whether it is joining a gym, hiring a certified personal trainer, or just making a healthy diet adjustment, this is when you have to start getting out of your comfort zone. If you approach your journey slowly and stay calm, this is a significant factor for long-term success.

EXAMPLE OF A SMART GOAL:

Specific	I will increase my daily activity by walking around the block for 20-30 minutes every morning.
Measurable	I will track my progress by using my Fitbit tracker and check my dashboard once every week.
Attainable	I will increase my daily activity by walking around the block 20-30 minutes at least four times a week.

Realistic	Daily movement will help me to lose weight and reduce my risk for diabetes type 2. It will also help me move more comfortably when I get together with my grandkids.
Timely	I will re-evaluate my goals in six to eight weeks and increase my walking time or make more adjustments to incorporate more physical activity into my lifestyle.

Below is a list of healthy tips to encourage you to make those small, impactful changes in your life. These minor beneficial adjustments will help you achieve your health and weight loss goals and, in the end, your overall success.

HOW TO START MAKING HEALTHIER CHOICES

1. Set a SMART goal. A Specific, Measurable, Attainable, Realistic, and Timely goal.
2. Choose to focus on one small healthy change at a time. Refrain from overwhelming yourself. Give yourself a reasonable amount of time to focus on making that one change before moving on.
3. Create small healthy habits you can keep and stay committed to.
4. Track your progress in whichever way you feel most comfortable. Some examples are taking before and after photos, taking body measurements, or using the number on

the scale. Use any method to give you an idea of where you were and where you are now.
5. Incorporate regular weekly exercise at least two to three times weekly. Start slowly and focus on moving your body as much as possible, even if you are just walking around the block. Walking as much as you can is a great place to start.
6. Drink lots of water and stay adequately hydrated throughout the day. Drinking 3-4 L of water a day helps keep your body from dehydrating and prevent other health problems caused by dehydration.
7. Stand up on your feet as much as possible throughout the day and try to avoid sitting for long periods of time. Using a standing desk is excellent for this.
8. Aim for a balanced whole-food diet and find an eating schedule that works for you without eating too close to bedtime.
9. Focus on the bigger picture and your long-term goals.
10. Stay positive and keep moving forward. Every day is a new opportunity to improve and live healthier and happier lives.

"DO THE ONE THING YOU THINK YOU CANNOT DO. FAIL AT IT. TRY AGAIN. DO BETTER THE SECOND TIME. THE ONLY PEOPLE WHO NEVER TUMBLE ARE THOSE WHO NEVER MOUNT THE HIGH WIRE. THIS IS YOUR MOMENT. OWN IT."

OPRAH WINFREY

5
MOVE YOUR BODY

In 2020, the World Health Organization changed their guidelines regarding recommended physical activity. As of 2023, the recommendation for physical activity is that all adults undertake 150–300 minutes of moderate-intensity, 75–150 minutes of vigorous-intensity, or some equivalent combination of moderate-intensity and vigorous-intensity aerobic physical activity per week.

"Among children and adolescents, an average of 60 minutes per day of moderate-to-vigorous intensity aerobic physical activity across the week provides health benefits" (Bull, 2020). Only 49% of adults 18 to 79 years of age living in Canada obtain at least 150 minutes of moderate to vigorous physical activity per week (Statistics Canada, custom tabulation, CHMS, Cycle 6 [2018 and 2019]). That percentage has continued to decrease as the years go by and technology progresses, more people are, as a result, adopting a more sedentary lifestyle.

For my journey, the gym became my sanctuary and working out became my therapy. The gym became a place I could connect with myself and work on myself. The gym became one of the only places I could zone out of the crazy world around me and focus on working on myself by myself for an hour or so. One of the most therapeutic activities I love to do when I am having a rough day is jam out to some old-school 90s and 2000 throwbacks and get a hardcore sweaty workout in. I always feel so much better afterwards.

Working out and fitness, in general, are the part of my weight loss journey in which I excelled and became extremely passionate about. Participating in daily exercise and finding my love for the gym has helped me find significant long-term success in my weight loss journey. Just like incorporating a healthy diet and a good sleep routine, regular exercise helps aid in long-term healthy weight loss. For most, regular exercise is an underrated tool that can help you excel on your weight loss journey, tone up your body, eliminate those last few stubborn pounds, and find long-term weight loss success.

Yes, it is true that you lose weight in the kitchen and get fit in the gym, but I also learned that you also see your true inner strengths and what you are truly capable of in the gym. I learned to love my body in ways I never imagined in my wildest dreams at the gym and saw my inner strengths in real-time action. Working out and, specifically, strength training gave me confidence that I never had before and that extra push I needed to succeed on my journey.

As I mentioned earlier, when I started my weight loss journey in 2014, I joined a local community centre gym where the average age was about eighty years old. For most beginners, just starting to work out, walking into a gym can be very intimidating. Since I became a trainer and have been involved in the fitness industry for quite some time now, I have noticed, unfortunately, that the fitness industry, in general, and most gyms are not geared to the average overweight person wanting or needing to get healthy. Instead, it is aimed toward a fit and healthy person getting fitter and healthier.

When I first became a fitness trainer, and still to this day, I never personally felt like the typical trainers in the fitness industry that you see at the gym. The stereotypical personal trainer has an excellent physique and has probably never been overweight or obese in their entire life. They may need help understanding the emotional side of a significant weight loss journey. There is a power of fitness beyond just moving your body and a dynamic factor that comes with someone's weight loss journey. A trainer needs to keep this in mind when building a workout program for a beginner focusing on the goal of weight loss.

CARDIOVASCULAR VS. STRENGTH TRAINING

When a beginner wants to start exercising for the first time, not knowing what to do, they come to a gym and head straight over to the treadmill or some other cardio machine. I have personally seen some people spend hours on cardio equipment, thinking that the longer they do it and the more they sweat, the more weight they will lose. That is a myth.

In the 90s, there was a marketing campaign in which the message was cardio, cardio, and more cardio for weight loss. Since then, many years have gone by and with all the progress in science and studies and through my personal and professional opinion, the best exercise routine is a combination of cardiovascular training, strength training, balance training, and flexibility training.

When it comes to working out, less is usually more. It is helpful to learn how to use exercise properly as a beneficial tool in your weight loss journey toolbox. Cardiovascular training, which includes walking or running on the treadmill, using an elliptical machine or stationary bike, should be used as a warm-up or after completing your strength training and on your active rest days. It would be best to incorporate strength training, at first, two to three times a week into your exercise routine for maximum success and then go from there.

EXAMPLES OF CARDIOVASCULAR AND STRENGTH EXERCISES:

Cardiovascular Exercises	Strength Exercises
Walking or Running	Squat
Swimming	Bench Press
Hiking	Plank
Dancing	Deadlift
Jump Rope	Push-Up

HIRE A CERTIFIED PERSONAL TRAINER

I am not just suggesting you hire a personal trainer because I am one, but a good certified personal trainer can be a valuable source to get you started on the right path for your weight loss or fitness journey. "Personal training results in a greater level of commitment to their journey from clients. 73% of participants using a Personal Trainer moved up a stage in action (e.g., contemplation to action; action to maintenance)" (McClaran, 2003).

It is like learning a new language when you start working out and learning to exercise correctly with proper form. It is the most intimidating step for most beginners. Most people starting their weight/fitness journey need help to figure out what to do when working out. Hiring a certified personal trainer helps with added accountability, extra motivation, an extra pair of eyes correcting your form, and someone to teach you how to maximize your workouts to achieve your fitness and/or weight loss goals.

Here are a few things to look out for when hiring a Personal Trainer. The first thing to ensure is that whomever you decide to hire has proper credentials from an accredited institution and some fitness certification or degree. Certified personal trainers should be insured and have some first-aid training. Many TikTok and Instagram influencers who post their workouts on social media are not certified personal trainers and they have yet to learn the science behind their actions. Ensure that the trainer you hire has proper fitness certification since working out can be risky and dangerous for you and your body if not done correctly.

It is also helpful if you connect with the certified personal trainer and are on the same page regarding achieving your fitness and weight loss goals. Keep in mind that there is an emotional side to most weight loss journeys. Weight loss can often be a sensitive subject for most men and women which is why they might, but not always, prefer a certified personal trainer of the same gender as them. A good certified personal trainer becomes your trainer, confidant, and coach. You need to feel comfortable with them and open up and trust your trainer on this journey.

> GLOBALLY, 1 IN 4 ADULTS DO NOT MEET THE GLOBAL RECOMMENDED LEVELS OF PHYSICAL ACTIVITY.
> (WORLD HEALTH ORGANIZATION, 2022)

CHOOSE A FORM OF EXERCISE YOU ENJOY

Enjoying what you do is beneficial for long-term success otherwise you will not last long on a fitness or weight loss journey. If you are one of those people who do not enjoy going to the gym, choose a form of daily movement you do enjoy. If you want to keep striving for continuous long-term success, there has to be an enjoyment factor. If you prefer dancing or participating in mixed martial arts or jiu-jitsu then do that. They are excellent forms of exercise. The most important factor for long-term success is to make sure you keep your body moving regularly by doing a form of exercise you enjoy.

For most beginners who are just starting to incorporate daily exercise without going to a gym, a great place to start is just walking. However, more is needed for significant weight loss or maintenance. That is where you need to get comfortable being uncomfortable and start incorporating other forms of training, such as strength and flexibility training. Incorporating strength training is very important for men and women to support their skeletal system, especially as you age and lose lean muscle mass naturally in a process called sarcopenia.

SARCOPENIA- DEFINED AS THE AGE-RELATED PROGRESSIVE LOSS OF MUSCLE MASS AND STRENGTH.

If you incorporate daily moderate to high-intensity exercise, it will take some time to see weight loss results, but they will come. If you start moving your body regularly and adjust your eating habits by making healthier food choices, you, too, can achieve your weight loss goals.

HOW TO INCORPORATE MORE MOVEMENT INTO YOUR DAILY LIFE

1. Include taking the stairs wherever possible. Whether you live in an apartment/condominium or work in a corporate building, try to take the stairs as much as possible instead of an elevator or escalator.
2. If you are driving somewhere, park further away from your destination. This is another easy way to add movement to your daily step count.
3. Try to stand as much as you can throughout the day. If you have a desk job, try incorporating a standing desk to help relieve back pain and improve posture.
4. Stretch daily and do a light exercise routine while watching TV.
5. If you are a gamer, use your gaming systems to play games which require body movement, including DDR and Wii Sports.
6. Dance! Dancing is a great way to get your body moving whether you are dancing in your kitchen to your favourite song or as part of your regular workouts like in a scheduled dance class. Dancing is excellent for the soul.
7. Use a wearable fitness tracker. Fitness trackers such as a Fitbit or Apple Watch help keep you accountable to your daily movement goals. With reminders and step counts, being more aware will push you that extra step and add extra motivation.

8. Avoid using food delivery apps. These apps are great for convenience, but it helps enable your lazy side as your orders get dropped off right to you without you having to move very much. If you want fast food, get up and go to the restaurant yourself. This helps to add extra daily movement.
9. Start cleaning up. It sounds annoying, but cleaning and doing chores around the house are a great way to incorporate more movement into your life.
10. Move your body every day. Please keep it simple, and move as much as you can. Our bodies were not made to sit all day.

"DON'T WAIT UNTIL YOU'VE REACHED YOUR GOAL TO BE PROUD OF YOURSELF. BE PROUD OF EVERY STEP YOU TAKE TOWARD REACHING THAT GOAL."

SIMONE BILES

6
DRINK UP AND STAY HYDRATED

Drinking enough water every day and staying properly hydrated is beneficial for many health-related reasons. I am sure you have heard countless times to drink more water. This is usually true, whether it comes from a doctor or your mother. Drinking enough water daily has many health benefits and is another excellent tool in your weight loss journey toolbox to help you achieve your health and weight loss goals.

According to a study by *Nutrition Reviews,* water comprises 75% of body weight in infants to 55% in older adults and is crucial for proper cell homeostasis and life. (Popkin, 2010). For the average adult male approximately 60% of their body is made up of water.

HOMEOSTASIS- DEFINED AS THE STATE OF BALANCE AMONG ALL THE BODY SYSTEMS NEEDED FOR THE BODY TO SURVIVE AND FUNCTION PROPERLY.

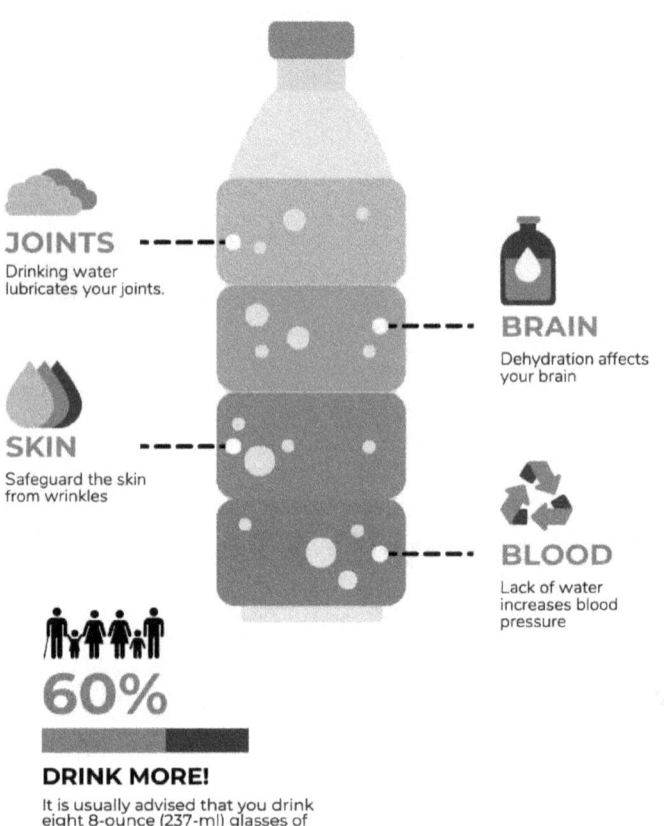

THE AVERAGE ADULT MALE HUMAN BODY COMPRISES AROUND 60% WATER.

Staying hydrated is necessary to help regulate body temperature, aid in digestion, flush bacteria from your body, help assist in healthy weight loss, protect organs and tissues, add moisture to your skin, and is, overall, very important for your general health.

As a picky eater, I know many people prefer to avoid drinking plain water, but there are easy ways to increase your water intake without drinking litres upon litres of plain tap water. It is beneficial for you to track your water intake and remember that water will also come from some of the foods you consume; for example, fruits and vegetables are great nutritious sources filled with water. Tracking your water intake will help you be more aware of how much water you drink throughout the day.

WATER AND WEIGHT LOSS

In order to adopt a healthier lifestyle and perhaps lose weight, water is an important tool. The great thing about water is it has zero calories. From a tap, it's also free. As a picky eater who never drank enough water, I had to learn how to increase my water intake as I entered my weight loss journey. It was a game-changer. It helped me to replenish what I lost during exercise as well as curbed my appetite. If I drink water before my meal, it signals to my brain my stomach is full and I eat less. Water is also in many fruits and vegetables we eat. Increasing my water intake helped with my skin and hair looking better than ever as well. It's also helpful to track how much you drink. Water is my drink of choice now. I normally drink 6-8 bottles or glasses of water a day. Personally, nothing is more refreshing than a cold bottle or glass of water. To add a little flavour without sugar, I also enjoy the odd Gatorade Zero after an intense workout. A study done in *Obesity* in 2008, showed that increases in drinking water were associated with significant weight loss and fat loss over time (Stookey, 2008).

There are countless benefits of staying properly hydrated. One such benefit is aiding in removing waste from the body. Water helps the kidneys filter out toxins and waste. When the body is dehydrated, the kidneys retain the fluid. That is why proper hydration is so important. Another benefit of water for weight loss is that without water, the body can not properly metabolize stored fats or carbohydrates. Drinking water and being adequately hydrated helps speed up your metabolism and, ultimately, helps burn more calories throughout the day while you are not eating.

If you have a weight loss goal, it is beneficial to trade in your sugary drinks, including high-sugar sports drinks, juices, and pop/soda, for a glass or bottle of water. Drinking water can help reduce your overall liquid calorie and total caloric intake. Juices, pop, and sports drinks are usually filled with sugar and empty calories that will not satisfy your thirst or hunger.

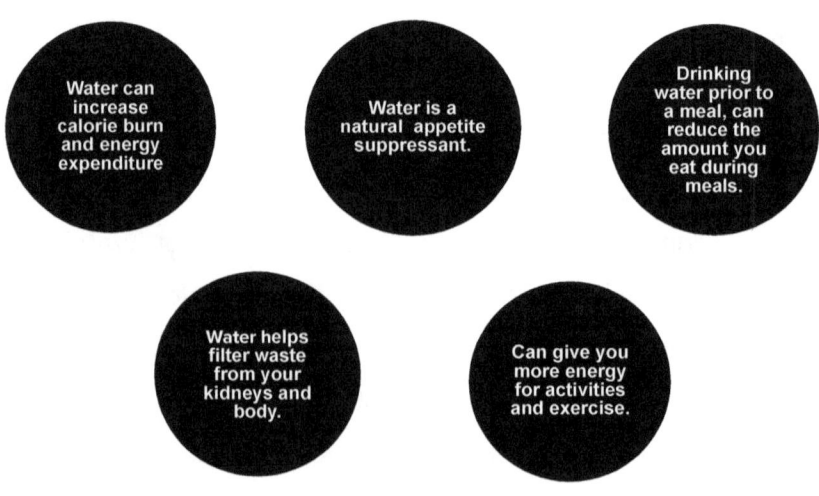

NOT A FAN OF STILL WATER?

As a fellow picky eater, I know some people are not such a fan of just plain water all the time. Some people might prefer flavour in their beverages, or you may prefer a carbonated drink over a still option. If you do not like plain still water, you can also consider other sugar and calorie-free options such as sparkling water, sparkling flavoured water, *Coke Zero*, *Sprite Zero*, *BioSteel*, *Gatorade Zero*, and *Nestea Zero*, just to name a few.

Consider, the next time you are thirsty, choosing a drink low in calories and containing little to no sugar. Maintaining proper hydration for someone on a weight loss journey is the most important attribute when choosing a beverage to hydrate you and keep your body flowing correctly. You do not want a highly caloric high-sugar drink full of empty calories that will not necessarily quench your thirst in the end.

Drinking enough water every day and staying properly hydrated will help you burn calories faster and speed up your metabolism to reach your weight loss goals more quickly. It is helpful to think of drinking more water as another tool in your toolbox of all your weight loss and healthy lifestyle tools, including a balanced, clean diet, regular exercise, a good sleep routine, and proper hydration. All these tools will help you achieve your weight loss goals.

HELPFUL TIPS TO INCREASE YOUR DAILY WATER INTAKE

1. Drink one glass of water when you wake up before eating breakfast.
2. Include drinking at least one glass of water with each meal.
3. Carry around a reusable water bottle so that it is easy to have water on hand. Use any water bottle filling station or sink to re-fill more easily.
4. Drink extra water when exercising. It is essential to keep your body temperature lower when you work out. Water and proper hydration help maintain a suitable body temperature and prevent overheating and dehydration.
5. Drink more water when it is warm or very humid outside.
6. Keep a glass of water at bedtime near your bedside.
7. Incorporate more soups and other liquid-rich meals, such as smoothies, stews, and curries, into your meal plans.
8. Include fruits and vegetables with high water content. You can also get some of your daily water consumption through foods such as berries, melons, celery, cucumber, and lettuce, to name a few.

"YOUR BODY IS SO HAPPY
WHEN YOU DRINK WATER."

CINDY CRAWFORD

7

LEARN TO LOVE YOURSELF

Self-love is the best love. The process of learning to truly love yourself is a complex multi-step journey that takes time, patience, self-discovery, and lots of self-care. This section of the journey is one of the more challenging parts. Some people will spend their whole lives trying to figure out this part. It is unfortunate, but most people, men and women, skinny or overweight, do not enjoy looking at themselves in a mirror or in photos because of their personal feelings toward themselves and their bodies.

The self-journey of learning to love yourself takes a lot of time, patience, self-motivation, body acceptance, self-confidence, and a much deeper dive into every aspect of your overall well-being, physically and mentally. It is not something you can do halfway or fake. You would only be negatively affecting yourself in the long term.

BODY ACCEPTANCE

Body acceptance, or accepting your own beauty, is one part of the process of learning to love yourself. It is a unique skill most people do not and never will have. We are the worst critics of our own bodies. The expectations that we should look some way are hard inner demons to fight with. It is sad, but the media tells us one way to look and dress. If you do not look like the norm, you are body-shamed or considered "different" looking. It takes time, but each day is a new opportunity to connect with yourself, be open to change, gain confidence, and learn to accept your beautiful body the way it is.

As I said at the beginning of the book, growing up in the 90s, I looked up to pop stars like Britney Spears, Christina Aguilera, Jessica Simpson, and Mandy Moore. The problem was that all of these girls were skinny and beautiful. That was hard since I did not see myself in any of them. It is challenging for any young kid, boy or girl, not to see themselves being represented.

On top of all that, I was body shamed and bullied about my weight from an early age. I was body shamed and called many names, from Free Willy (referencing the 90s movie about a whale) to Danny Devito to being called "fat" right to my face. The first time I remember clearly being body shamed was when I was about ten years old. My self-esteem was stomped on and broken down by a male acquaintance.

Even more than two decades later, I remember it like it was yesterday. I was at overnight camp hanging out with some of my male friends at rest hour, and a mutual male friend came right up to me, pointed at me, and yelled, "You are fat!" He laughed hysterically and ran away. Perhaps, he thought he was being funny or trying to be cool, but those three words broke my self-esteem for many years to come. I remember being very emotional and hurt. It was hard for a ten-year-old, vulnerable girl to hear. It was the first time I felt external judgement due to my weight and unfortunately, it was not the last.

Learning to love myself and my body has been a long and complex internal process that came along with adopting a healthy lifestyle and my significant weight loss. Learning the practice of daily self-love, self-care, and believing wholeheartedly in myself has helped me let go of my past with the inner hate I developed against my own body. Learning to love yourself is a skill, that once it is developed, you will want to keep working on it at every opportunity you get.

BELIEVE IN YOURSELF

In the words of my fellow Torontonian, Drake, "I started from the bottom, and now I am here." Usually, that is where this journey begins for most people, the bottom. Healthy weight loss is a personal journey you have to be ready for, you have to believe in yourself, and only you can be the one to do the hard work. When you are in the contemplation stage of action, it is important not to feel pressured or forced by anybody else to start this journey or it will most likely not work out long-term.

During my journey, I started reciting to myself positive affirmations every morning and night. *I am beautiful. I am strong. I will get through anything thrown my way today. Repeat.* Positive affirmations are phrases that start with "I" that you can say out loud or in your head to affirm yourself. Repeating these phrases over and over helps improve your self-esteem, self-confidence, and helps overcome self-sabotage. The most helpful affirmations are positive, in the present tense, and personal. Saying them aloud or in your head are practical ways to clear negative thoughts in stressful situations.

EXAMPLES OF POSITIVE AFFIRMATIONS

- I am beautiful.
- I am strong.
- I am worthy.
- I am proud of myself.
- I am healthy.
- I am full of gratitude.
- I am enough.
- I can get through anything.
- I am brave.
- I will be present in every moment.
- I believe in myself.
- I am unstoppable.

BE GRATEFUL FOR WHAT YOU HAVE

Another part of the process of learning to love yourself is being grateful for and accepting what you already have and who you are as an individual. Everybody is beautiful in their own unique way and you will realize you have more to be thankful for than you think. Some people find it very useful to start a gratitude journal to track daily what they are grateful for. It is a helpful way to be aware and retrain your mindset to focus on the positive aspects of your life. Being aware of your daily personal actions and your body physically and mentally is very important in the journey of self-love.

Every day it is so important to remember that you are alive, healthy, and beautiful. Also, if you are reading this book, you are on the right track and intend to positively change your life in the right direction. It all comes down to believing in yourself, knowing you can do anything you put your mind to, and seeing yourself as your biggest fan rather than your worst critic. Love your body. You are beautiful just the way you are.

HOW TO IMPROVE YOUR SELF CONFIDENCE

1. Keep your thinking positive and retrain your mindset to remove the negative thoughts. Focus on what you like or love about yourself rather than what you do not.
2. Practice some form of self-care daily. Recognize, be aware, and accept how you are feeling every day. It is normal to have bad days and good days. Everyone does.

3. Keep positive people around you and people who lift you and do not put you down.
4. Start getting comfortable saying no. It is okay to say no if you do not want to do something or are uncomfortable. Know your boundaries and, when saying "no", be polite, be firm, and do not be overly apologetic. Put yourself first, and don't be a people pleaser.
5. Be kind to yourself. Most people are their own worst critics, but you should believe in yourself and see your beauty in the world.
6. Do not compare yourself or your journey to others. Everyone is on their own journey and there should be no competition.
7. Learn to accept change and get comfortable out of your comfort zone. Growth only happens when you are out of your comfort zone.
8. Create and practice daily self-affirmations. Start your affirmations with "I" or "My" and keep your statements positive, present, and personal. Examples include *I am strong, I am beautiful, I am fierce, and I will conquer the day.*
9. Participate in regular daily activities and take care of your body. Learn that the best investment you can make is in your health and overall well-being.
10. Set your goals and crush them. Self-confidence is learning to connect with yourself deeper and shifting your mindset to a different and positive way of thinking.

"THE MINUTE YOU LEARN TO LOVE YOURSELF, YOU WON'T WANT TO BE ANYONE ELSE."

RIHANNA

8

SELF CARE: MIND, BODY & SOUL

Adopting and living a balanced healthy lifestyle is a great way to improve your overall well-being. Self-care is the practice of looking after oneself and prioritizing one's mental health and physical well-being. Daily self-care is important when someone is healthy with no illnesses, but self-care becomes essential when disease occurs.

Daily self-care has many benefits including, but not limited to, preventing diseases, improving your mental health and overall better quality of life. Some people think that examples of self-care include getting a manicure/pedicure, going for a massage, going on vacation, or working out, just to name a few. They are not wrong. Self-care also includes getting a good night's sleep and even a hot shower. Self-care is about doing whatever you enjoy and what makes you feel good. A lack of self-care is self-neglect, which means you do not take care of yourself mentally or physically.

SELF-MONITORING

Self-monitoring is a helpful way to keep you accountable to yourself on your weight loss journey. Using fitness wearables such as a Fitbit, or Apple Watch, or even using a scale helps monitor your progress on your journey. A study that was done by *Retrofit* between 2011-2015, showed that self-monitoring behaviours, such as self-weigh-ins, tracking daily step counts, high-intensity activity, and consistent food logging, were significant predictors of weight change at six months.

In this study, weighing in three times or more per week, having a minimum of 60 highly active minutes per week, food logging for three days or more per week, and having a higher percentage of weeks with five or more food logs increased overall weight-loss success. (Painter, 2017)

MANAGING STRESS LEVELS

Stress is something everybody deals with to some extent. Stress has been known to do mysterious and unexplainable things to people's bodies. Stress has been known to cause gastric problems and could even cause eating disorders such as starvation or binging. A daily practice of self-care will help with how you and your body react to daily stressors.

When you are stressed, the body releases the hormone cortisol. Cortisol is the stress hormone, and increased levels can do many things to the body, including increasing sugar levels, which can ultimately lead to weight gain. Incorporating stress management techniques such as guided meditation, breath work, participating in daily physical exercise, adopting a healthy diet, limiting social media use, and connecting with others are great ways to manage stress levels and your body's reaction to stress.

THE EFFECTS OF STRESS AND WEIGHT GAIN:

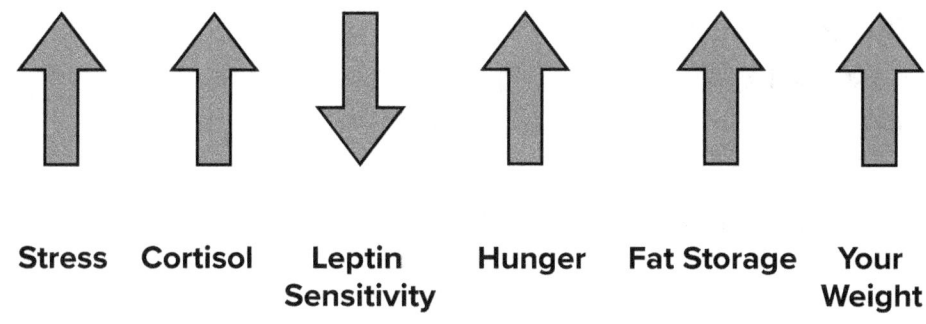

Stress   Cortisol   Leptin   Hunger   Fat Storage   Your
**   Sensitivity   Weight**

It is also good to keep an eye out for others you care about dealing with excessive stress or anxiety-related issues. Look out for the signs like uncontrollable worry, panic attacks, or a person being overwhelmed by stress. In these cases, connecting them with mental health resources might be helpful.

SLEEP IS ESSENTIAL

Adopting a consistent healthy sleep routine is another underrated tool in your weight loss toolbox that many people should take more advantage of. I am sure you have heard before that you should get 7-9 hours of good restful sleep every night for proper bodily function and all the health benefits you get from a healthy sleep routine. I understand it is not accessible or attainable for everyone, but the more sleep you get, the better.

Many benefits come from getting a good sleep routine, from how your body recovers after working out, to increasing the speed of your metabolism. People with poor sleep have been linked to a slower metabolism and a higher BMI. Depending on your stage in life, if you have newborns or overnight shifts, it is tough to get into a good sleep routine, but it is something to prioritize in your lifestyle to achieve weight loss goals. A good sleep routine is vital in a healthy weight loss journey and could be the key to losing those last few stubborn pounds.

TAKING CARE OF YOUR MENTAL HEALTH

When practicing healthy self-care, taking care of your mental health is just as important as looking after your physical health. It is important to prioritize both your physical and psychological well-being. It can be sometimes helpful for you to participate in traditional or unconventional therapy since prioritizing your mental health is vital to your overall self-care and lifestyle change.

Making those small and healthy daily changes to your lifestyle to improve your mental health will help you stay as positive as possible during this bumpy personal weight loss journey that can sometimes get emotional or frustrating. Participating in regular physical activity and keeping your mindset positive are constructive ways to improve your overall mental health. A positive attitude also helps bring positive things in life to occur.

The acts of healthy self-care will look different for everyone, as everybody's journey is different and unique. Depending on your current lifestyle, family status, and the activities you enjoy that make you feel good, there are many ways to prioritize your physical and mental health. Participating in daily self-care and prioritizing your mental and physical health will help manage stress levels and how your body reacts to daily stressors. It will also keep your body functioning properly and helps improve your mental and physical health.

Healthy self-care can be as easy as taking a warm shower, getting a good night's sleep, or getting in a sweaty workout. Every day is a new opportunity to better yourself and invest in your mental and physical health. Aim for the stars and strive to be your best self.

TEN WAYS TO PRACTICE DAILY SELF-CARE

1. Make your overall personal happiness a priority. Building a solid foundation for yourself is helpful in your other relationships and daily life. Remember that each day is a new chance to focus on your happiness.
2. Consume healthy balanced meals and hydrate properly by drinking water and zero sugar alternatives.
3. Stay connected socially. Being socially connected is crucial for your positive mindset and overall health.

4. Make sleep a priority in your daily routine. Aim for 7-9 hours of good restful sleep.
5. Make SMART goals and work hard to strive for them.
6. Try a relaxing activity such as yoga, meditation, breath work or swimming.
7. Get regular physical activity. Aim for 30 minutes a day of moderate-vigorous physical activity.
8. Get a dog. They provide unconditional love, help you with self-care, and get your daily step count in by taking them for multiple daily walks.
9. Get outside and enjoy some fresh air every day, even briefly. For example, go for a walk around the block or walk to a friend or family member's house.
10. Stay as positive as possible and keep moving forward. If you fall off, get back up and keep going strong.

"THE MOST IMPORTANT RELATIONSHIP IN YOUR LIFE IS THE ONE WITH YOURSELF."

DIANE VON FURSTENBERG

9
CONCLUSION

As I have continued to say throughout the book, everybody's weight loss journey will be a different experience. Something that personally worked for me to achieve my weight loss and fitness goals does not necessarily mean it will work for you and achieving your weight loss goals. It is pretty clear that in order to maintain long-term weight loss, a very restrictive diet won't work. Life is too short. Any healthy long-term weight loss journey should be a balanced lifestyle approach. You need to put 100% into your diet, 100% into exercise, and 100% with a positive mindset.

If you go into your weight loss journey with a healthy lifestyle approach and a positive mindset, you too can get the body you have always dreamed of and keep off your weight loss goals long-term. Everybody with a fantastic personality can use a beautiful body if they are willing to work hard. If I could lose over 100 pounds and keep it off for almost a decade by changing my daily habits without eating a salad, you can too.

As a nationally certified personal trainer with multiple fitness specializations and someone who personally went through a significant weight loss journey, the most successful approach to long-term weight loss success is a balanced healthy lifestyle and overall consistency. This is the only approach to weight loss that you never have to restrict yourself from the good stuff in life. I still enjoy eating pizza, chicken wings, sushi, and all my other favourites, but in moderation and not every day or week. The magic combination of a healthy balanced lifestyle consists of a balanced diet, regular exercise, good sleep, and daily self-care to manage stress levels. Any weight loss and fitness lifestyle is a journey that does not matter if you are eighteen or eighty. It does not have an end date.

No matter who you are, everyone needs to prioritize their mental and physical health. You do not need to starve yourself or only eat salads all day to achieve your weight loss goals and keep them off for years. To most overweight/obese people, losing a significant amount of weight loss is highly overwhelming. This is why most people fail at achieving their goals or do not even try. I am here to tell you that if you break it down into small healthy changes and believe in yourself, you, too, can turn your health and overall well-being around.

As I mentioned earlier, be aware of the weight loss quick fixes and fads you see on the market or on social media. Also, some of these quick weight loss fixes you see on social media are only sometimes healthy for you and can sometimes do more damage than good. Do your research, it is not recommended to find your health and fitness advice on social media platforms such as TikTok or Instagram.

Ultimately, weight loss comes down to calories in versus calories out. There is no crazy science to it, but most overweight/obese people find it one of the hardest things to commit to and accomplish. Unfortunately, some people will be trying to lose weight using quick fixes or fads their entire lives because they are looking for quick fixes and are unwilling to commit to doing the hard work for themselves and making an actual healthy lifestyle change. On average, ninety percent of people fail multiple times at trying to lose weight and, most of the time, give up trying to lose weight and be healthier for good. Being fit and healthy is hard, but so is being overweight and unhealthy. So which "hard" do you choose?

A healthy lifestyle combines a clean, balanced diet, regular exercise, and a positive mindset. It is important to retrain your brain to turn negative thoughts into positive ones and keep moving forward. This process does not happen overnight, but with patience, time, and hard work, you will achieve the weight loss goals you worked so hard for and keep the pounds off long-term.

Your success in any weight loss journey comes down to you, and you are the only person who can do the hard work required to go through a healthy weight loss journey successfully. Hiring a certified personal trainer is a tool that is extremely helpful on your journey to keep you accountable and lead you in the right direction. Still, in the end, you are the only one who can change your habits and do the hard work to achieve success.

If approached correctly, this journey is not just about weight loss and fitting into your old jeans again but a journey of self-discovery, self-love, and finding your true inner strength. You will learn a lot about yourself. Your age does not matter. You will shock and impress yourself. You do not even need to eat a salad, I promise.

Go one step at a time and take tiny baby steps forward. You will get to the finish line and change your mindset for good. I know many people look for a quick fix because they think it is easier, but your goal should not just be losing weight for a particular function, such as a wedding or a high school reunion. You should want to maintain a healthy weight at any age for your health and well-being. You have to believe in yourself and get comfortable with being uncomfortable. Find a way that works for you and you can also lose a significant amount of weight without eating just salads and/or starving yourself.

Do not wait until tomorrow. Start your weight loss journey today by making minor adjustments to your lifestyle to adopt a healthier, balanced approach. Believe in yourself and take that first leap of faith into caring for yourself and your overall health. Stay positive on this journey, and stay strong! If you fall off, get up, dust yourself off and keep moving forward. This is not a sprint. It is a marathon for the rest of your life. Enjoy the ride.

If I can do it, so can you. Take a big deep breath and believe that you can do anything you set your mind to. Take that one small step forward, do not overwhelm yourself and never stop. You will shock yourself where you are in a year from now. You are the only one who can do the hard work that has to be done, so believe in yourself and learn to love yourself. Each day is a new opportunity to better yourself and achieve your goals.

Just believe in yourself and stay strong.

You've got this!

"DOUBT IS A KILLER. YOU JUST HAVE TO KNOW WHO YOU ARE AND WHAT YOU STAND FOR."

JENNIFER LOPEZ

PART II: HEALTHY RECIPES FOR PICKY EATERS
(NO SALADS INCLUDED)

HEALTHY RECIPES FOR PICKY EATERS

GRILLED CHICKEN BREAST WITH ROASTED VEGETABLES

BAKED SALMON WITH ASPARAGUS

HEALTHY CAULIFLOWER RICE WITH SAUTÉED SHRIMP

BROILED PORK CHOPS WITH STEAMED BROCCOLI

SCRAMBLED EGGS AND SAUSAGE

TURKEY MEATBALLS WITH ZUCCHINI NOODLES

BLACKENED TUNA STEAK WITH AVOCADO SALSA

FAJITA CHICKEN BOWL WITH CAULIFLOWER RICE

LOW CARB CHILLI WITH GROUND BEEF/CHICKEN

GRILLED SHRIMP SKEWERS WITH BELL PEPPERS AND ONIONS

EGGPLANT LASAGNA WITH GROUND TURKEY

SPICY CHICKEN AND VEGETABLE STIR FRY

BAKED COD WITH GARLIC BUTTER AND LEMON

ROASTED CHICKEN THIGHS WITH BRUSSELS SPROUTS

CHICKEN FRIED RICE

GRILLED CHICKEN BREAST WITH ROASTED VEGETABLES

Calories: 374cal, Protein: 45g, Carbohydrate: 8g, Fat: 18g
Prep time: 15 minutes, Cook time: 25 minutes, Serving: 4

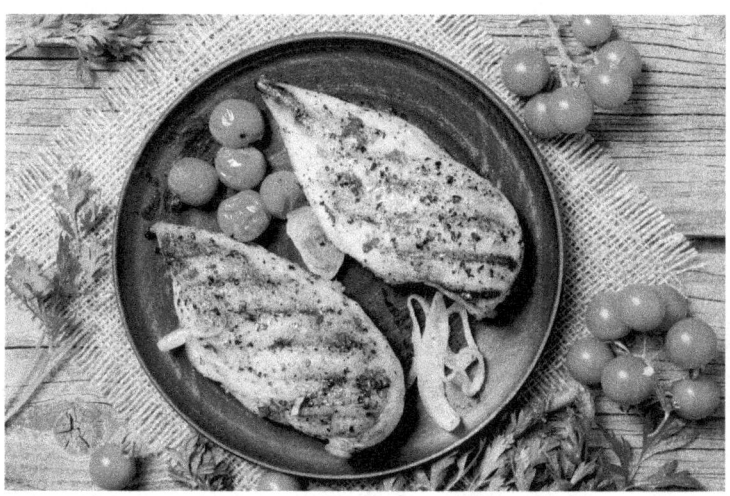

Ingredients:
- 4 boneless, skinless chicken breasts
- 1 medium zucchini, sliced
- 2 cups broccoli florets
- 1 yellow bell pepper, sliced
- 1 red onion, sliced
- 2 tbsp olive oil
- 1 tsp garlic powder
- 1 tsp dried oregano
- 1 tsp dried basil
- Salt and crushed pepper, to taste

Instructions:
- Preheat oven to 400F (200°C). Place sliced vegetables on a large baking sheet. Drizzle the olive oil and sprinkle it with garlic powder, oregano, basil, salt, and crushed pepper. Toss vegetables to coat.
- Bake for 23-25 minutes or until tender vegetables are lightly browned. While vegetables are roasting, preheat the grill to medium-high heat. Sprinkle the chicken breasts with salt and crushed pepper.
- Grill chicken for 6-8 minutes for each side or until cooked. Serve chicken with roasted vegetables.

BAKED SALMON WITH ASPARAGUS

Calories: 330cal, Protein: 37g, Carbohydrate: 5g, Fat: 18g
Prep time: 10 minutes, Cook time: 15 minutes, Serving: 4

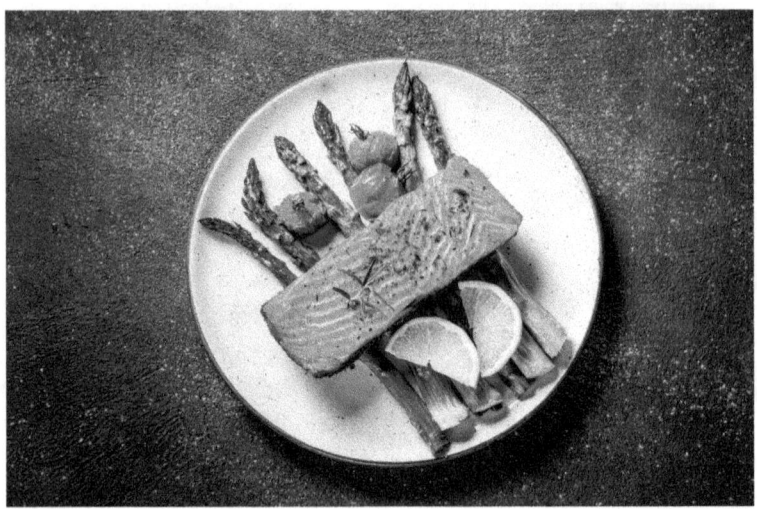

Ingredients:
- 4 salmon fillets
- 1 pound of asparagus, trimmed
- 2 tbsp olive oil
- 2 cloves garlic, minced
- 1 tbsp lemon juice
- Salt and crushed pepper, to taste

Instructions:
- Preheat oven to 400F
- Place salmon fillets and asparagus in a single layer on a baking sheet. Drizzle the olive oil and sprinkle it with garlic, lemon juice, salt, and pepper.
- Bake for 13-15 minutes or until salmon is cooked and asparagus is tender.
- Serve immediately.

HEALTHY CAULIFLOWER RICE WITH SAUTÉED SHRIMP

Calories: 221cal, Protein: 28g, Carbohydrates: 7g, Fat: 9g
Prep time: 10 minutes, Cook time: 15 minutes, Serving: 4

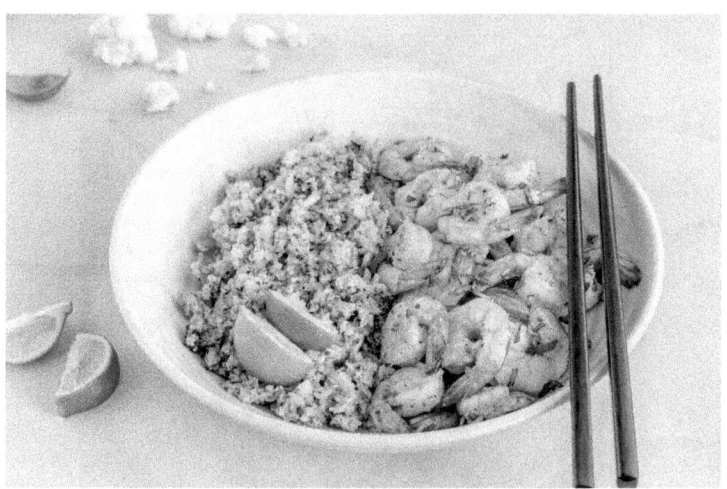

Ingredients:
- 1 head of cauliflower, grated
- 1 pound of shrimp, peeled and deveined
- 2 tbsp. of olive oil
- 2 cloves garlic, minced
- 1 tbsp. of ginger, grated
- 1 tbsp. soy sauce
- Salt and crushed pepper, to taste

Instructions:
- Put the non-stick skillet over medium heat. Add olive oil, garlic, and ginger to the skillet and sauté for 1-2 minutes. Add shrimp to the skillet and cook for 3-4 minutes or until pink. Remove shrimp from the skillet and set aside.
- Add grated cauliflower to the same skillet and sauté for 4-5 minutes or until tender. Add soy sauce and salt and pepper to taste. Stir in cooked shrimp.
- Serve immediately.

BROILED PORK CHOPS WITH STEAMED BROCCOLI

Calories: 336cal, Protein: 22g, Carbohydrate: 8g, Fat: 24g
Prep time: 10 minutes, Cook time: 20 minutes, Serving: 4

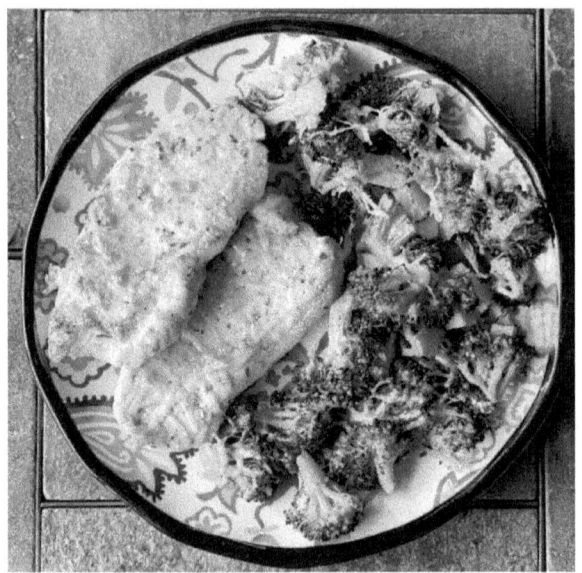

Ingredients:
- 4 bone-in pork chops
- 1 tbsp olive oil
- 1 tsp garlic powder
- 1 tsp dried thyme
- 1 tsp paprika
- Salt and crushed pepper, to taste
- 1 pound of broccoli florets

Instructions:
- Preheat the broiler on high heat—season pork chops with olive oil, garlic powder, thyme, paprika, salt, and pepper. Place pork chops on a broiler pan and broil for 8-10 minutes per side or until cooked.
- While cooking, steam the broccoli for 5-7 minutes or until tender.
- Serve pork chops with steamed broccoli.

SCRAMBLED EGGS AND SAUSAGE

Calories: 337cal, Protein: 18g, Carbohydrate: 1g, Fat: 29g
Prep time: 5 minutes, Cook time: 10 minutes, Serving: 2

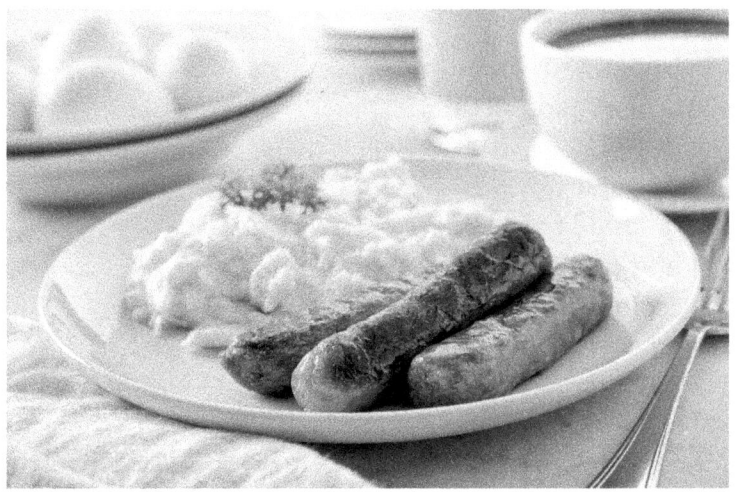

Ingredients:
- 4 large eggs
- 4 breakfast sausage links, sliced
- 2 tbsp. of butter
- Salt and crushed pepper, to taste

Instructions:
- Heat a large skillet over medium heat. Add sausage links to the skillet and cook until browned. Remove sausage from the skillet and set aside. Crack eggs into a bowl and whisk with salt and pepper.
- Melt two tbsp butter in the same skillet over medium heat. Pour whisked eggs into the skillet and scramble until cooked through. Add cooked sausage to the skillet and stir to combine.
- Serve immediately.

TURKEY MEATBALLS WITH ZUCCHINI NOODLES

Calories: 355cal, Protein: 36g, Carbohydrate: 10g, Fat: 19g
Prep time: 15 minutes, Cook time: 25 minutes, Serving: 4

Ingredients:
- 1 pound of ground turkey
- ¼ cup of almond flour
- 1 egg
- 1 tbsp. garlic powder
- 1 tbsp. dried basil
- Salt and crushed pepper, to taste
- 4 zucchinis, spiralized
- 1 tbsp. of olive oil
- 1 cup of marinara sauce

Instructions:
- Preheat oven to 375F. Mix ground turkey, almond flour, egg, garlic powder, dried basil, salt, and pepper in a large bowl—form the mixture into meatballs.
- Put meatballs on the baking sheet and bake for 20-25 minutes or until cooked. While baking, heat one tbsp olive oil in a large skillet over medium heat. Add spiralized zucchini to the skillet and sauté for 3-4 minutes or until tender.
- Pour marinara sauce over the zucchini noodles and stir to combine. Serve turkey meatballs over zucchini noodles.

BLACKENED TUNA STEAK WITH AVOCADO SALSA

Calories: 401cal, Protein: 42g, Carbohydrate: 11g, Fat: 21g
Prep time: 10 minutes, Cook time: 10 minutes, Serving: 2

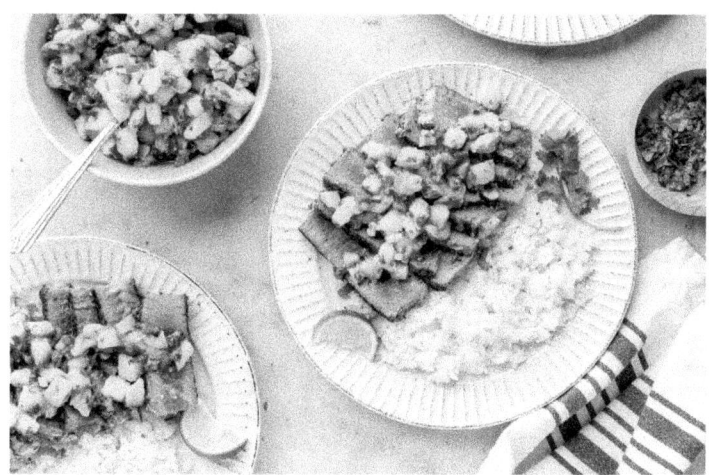

Ingredients:
- 2 (6 oz. each weight) tuna steaks
- 1 tbsp smoked paprika
- 1 tsp cumin
- 1 tsp garlic powder
- ½ tsp salt
- ¼ tsp cayenne pepper
- 1 tbsp. of olive oil
- 100g avocado, diced
- ¼ cup diced red onion
- ¼ cup chopped fresh cilantro
- 1 lime, juiced

Instructions:
- Combine the smoked paprika with cumin, garlic powder, salt, and cayenne pepper to create a spice rub. Rub the tuna steaks sides with the spice rub. Heat one tbsp olive oil in a large skillet over medium-high heat.
- Once hot, add tuna steaks to the skillet and cook for 2-3 minutes per side or until blackened on the outside and cooked to your desired doneness. While the tuna is cooking, make the avocado salsa by combining diced avocado, red onion, cilantro, and lime juice in a small bowl.
- Season with salt to taste. Once the tuna is done, transfer it to a plate and top it with the avocado salsa. Serve immediately.

FAJITA CHICKEN BOWL WITH CAULIFLOWER RICE

Calories: 260cal, Protein: 26g, Carbohydrate: 12g, Fat: 12g
Prep time: 10 minutes, Cook time: 20 minutes, Serving: 4

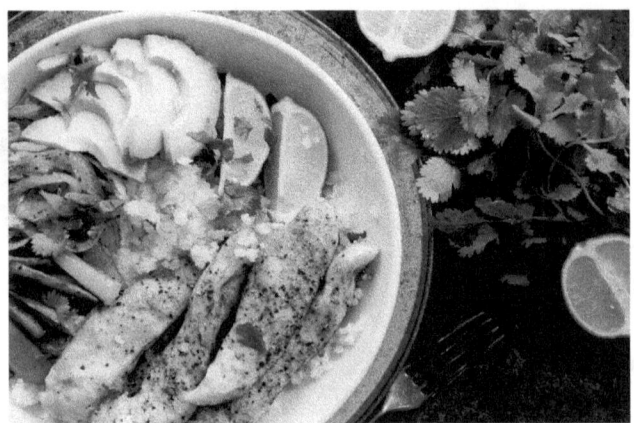

Ingredients:
- 1 pound of chicken breast, sliced
- 1 green bell pepper, sliced
- 1 onion, sliced
- 1 tbsp. of olive oil
- 2 tbsp. fajita seasoning
- Salt and crushed pepper, to taste
- One head of cauliflower, grated into rice
- 2 tbsp. of butter
- ¼ cup chopped fresh cilantro
- Lime wedges for serving

Instructions:
- In a non-stick skillet, heat olive oil over medium-high heat. Add chicken, bell peppers, and onion to the skillet and sprinkle with fajita seasoning, salt, and pepper. Cook until chicken is browned and vegetables are tender, stirring occasionally.
- While chicken and vegetables are cooking, grate the cauliflower into rice using a food processor or cheese grater. Melt two tbsp butter in a separate skillet over medium heat. Add cauliflower rice to the skillet and sauté for 5-7 minutes or until tender.
- Season cauliflower rice with salt and pepper to taste. Divide cauliflower rice among four bowls and top with fajita chicken and vegetables. Garnish with chopped cilantro and serve with lime wedges.

LOW CARB CHILLI WITH GROUND BEEF/CHICKEN

Calories: 200cal, Protein: 25g, Carbohydrate: 7g, Fat: 8g
Prep time: 10 minutes, Cook time: 40 minutes, Serving: 6

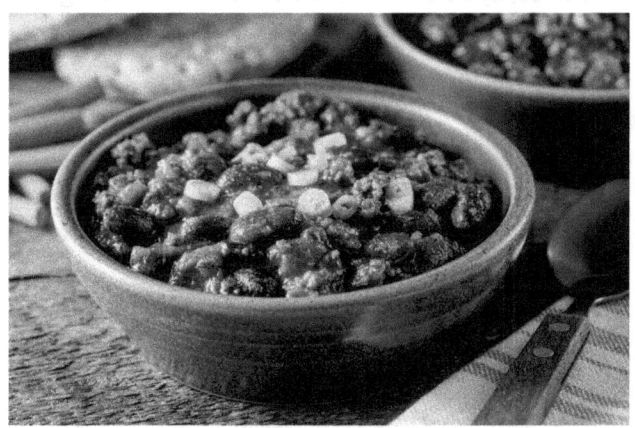

Ingredients:
- 1 pound of ground beef or chicken
- 1 onion, diced
- 3 cloves garlic, minced
- 1 red bell pepper, diced
- 1 jalapeño pepper, diced
- 2 tbsp chilli powder
- 1 tbsp ground cumin
- 1 tsp smoked paprika
- ½ tsp salt
- ¼ tsp black pepper
- 1 can (15 oz weight) of diced tomatoes
- 1 cup of beef broth
- 1 tbsp. of olive oil
- Sour cream & shredded cheddar cheese for serving

Instructions:
- Heat one tbsp olive oil in a non-stick pot over medium-high heat. Add ground meat to the pot and cook until browned. Add onion, garlic, bell peppers, and jalapeño pepper to the pot and cook until vegetables are tender.
- Add chilli powder, cumin, smoked paprika, salt, and black pepper to the pot and stir until well combined. Add diced tomatoes and beef broth to the pot and boil. Decrease the stove heat and simmer for 30 minutes, stirring occasionally.
- If desired, serve hot with a dollop of sour cream and shredded cheddar cheese.

GRILLED SHRIMP SKEWERS WITH BELL PEPPERS AND ONIONS

Calories: 250cal, Protein: 23g, Carbohydrate: 8g, Fat: 14g
Prep time: 20 minutes, Cook time: 10 minutes, Serving: 4

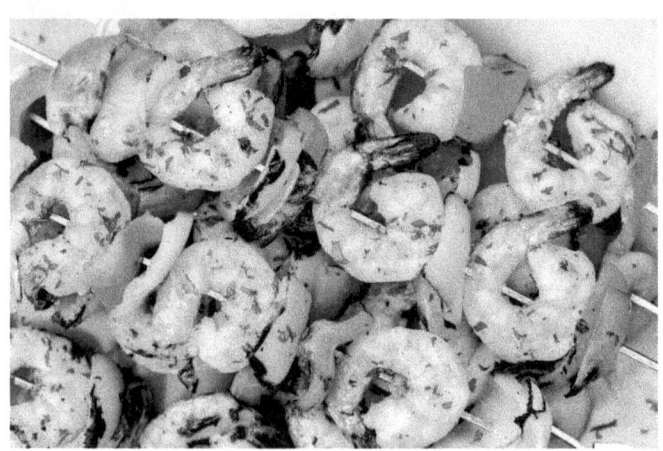

Ingredients:
- 1 pound of large shrimp, peeled and deveined
- 1 red bell pepper, seedless and cut into chunks
- 1 red onion, cut into chunks
- 4 tbsp olive oil
- 1 tbsp smoked paprika
- 1 tsp garlic powder
- ½ tsp salt
- ¼ tsp black pepper
- 8 wooden skewers, soaked in water for thirty minutes

Instructions:
- Preheat the grill to medium-high heat—thread shrimp, bell peppers, and onions onto skewers, alternating between each ingredient. Whisk the olive oil with smoked paprika, garlic powder, salt, and crushed pepper in a bowl.
- Brush skewers with the spice mixture. Grill skewers for 2-3 minutes per side or until shrimp are pink and cooked through.
- Serve hot.

EGGPLANT LASAGNA WITH GROUND TURKEY

Calories: 350cal, Protein: 36g, Carbohydrate: 11g, Fat: 18g
Prep time: 20 minutes, Cook time: 45 minutes, Serving: 6

Ingredients:
- 2 large eggplants, sliced lengthwise into 1/4-inch-thick pieces
- 1 pound of ground turkey
- 1 cup onion, chopped
- 3 cloves garlic, minced
- 1 can (15 oz weight) of crushed tomatoes
- 2 tbsp tomato paste
- 1 tsp dried basil
- 1 tsp dried oregano
- 1 tsp salt
- ¼ tsp black pepper
- 2 cups low-fat ricotta cheese
- ¼ cup grated Parmesan cheese
- 1 egg
- 2 cups shredded mozzarella cheese

Instructions:
- Preheat oven to 375°F. Arrange the baking sheet with parchment paper and place eggplant slices on top. Roast in the oven for 15-20 minutes or until tender. Put the non-stick skillet over medium-high heat, and brown the ground turkey with chopped onion and garlic.
- Stir in crushed tomatoes, tomato paste, dried basil, dried oregano, salt, and black pepper. Simmer for 10-15 minutes or until thickened. Mix the low-fat ricotta cheese with Parmesan cheese and egg in a bowl.
- In a 9x13-inch baking dish, layer the roasted eggplant slices, turkey tomato sauce, and ricotta cheese mixture. Repeat layers until all ingredients are used up. Top with shredded mozzarella cheese.
- Cover the baking dish with a foil sheet and bake in the oven for 23-25 minutes. Remove the foil and bake for 13-15 minutes.
- Let cool for 5-10 minutes before serving.

SPICY CHICKEN AND VEGETABLE STIR FRY

Calories: 329cal, Protein: 35g, Carbohydrate: 9g, Fat: 17g
Prep time: 15 minutes, Cook time: 15 minutes, Serving: 4

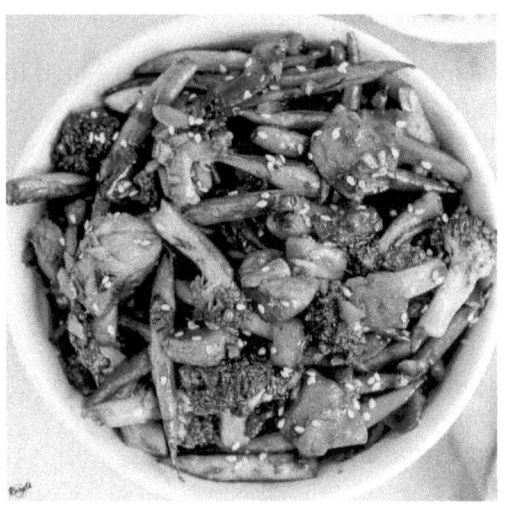

Ingredients:
- 1 pound chicken breasts (without bone and skin) cut into thin strips
- 2 cups mixed vegetables (carrot, onions, and broccoli)
- 2 tbsp olive oil
- 2 cloves garlic, minced
- 1 tbsp soy sauce
- 1 tsp Sriracha sauce
- ½ tsp ground ginger
- ½ tsp salt
- ¼ tsp black pepper

Instructions:
- Heat two tbsp olive oil in a wok over medium-high heat. Add chicken strips to the skillet and cook until browned on all sides. Add mixed vegetables with minced garlic to the skillet and stir for 7 minutes or until vegetables are tender-crisp.
- Mix the soy sauce with Sriracha sauce, ground ginger, salt, and black pepper in a small bowl. Pour the ginger sauce over the chicken and vegetables in the skillet and stir until well combined.
- Cook for 2-3 minutes or until the sauce has thickened.
- Serve immediately.

BAKED COD WITH GARLIC BUTTER AND LEMON

Calories: 245cal, Protein: 31g, Carbohydrate: 1g, Fat: 13g
Prep time: 10 minutes, Cook time: 15 minutes, Serving: 4

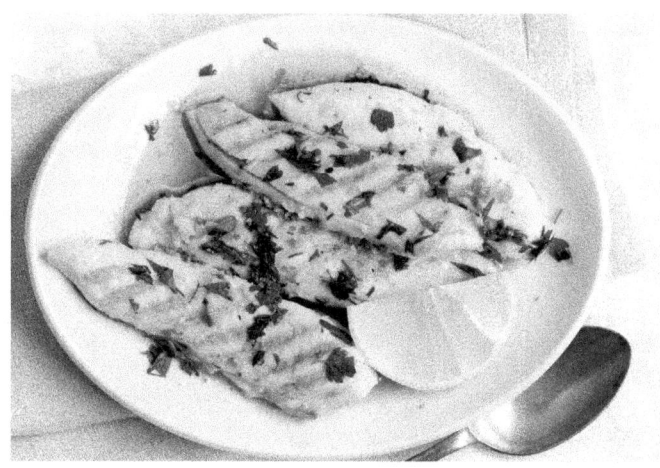

Ingredients:
- 4 cod fillets (6 oz each weight)
- ¼ cup unsalted butter melted
- 3 cloves garlic, minced
- 2 tbsp lemon juice
- ½ tsp salt
- ¼ tsp black pepper
- Lemon wedges and chopped parsley for serving

Instructions:
- Preheat oven to 400F—place cod fillets in a single layer in a baking dish. Whisk together melted butter, garlic, lemon juice, salt, and black pepper in a small bowl. Pour the butter mixture over the cod fillets.
- Bake for 12-15 minutes until fish is cooked and flakes easily with a fork.
- Serve hot with lemon wedges and chopped parsley.

ROASTED CHICKEN THIGHS WITH BRUSSELS SPROUTS

Calories: 336cal, Protein: 20g, Carbohydrate: 10g, Fat: 24g
Perp time: 10 minutes, Cook time: 45 minutes, Serving: 4

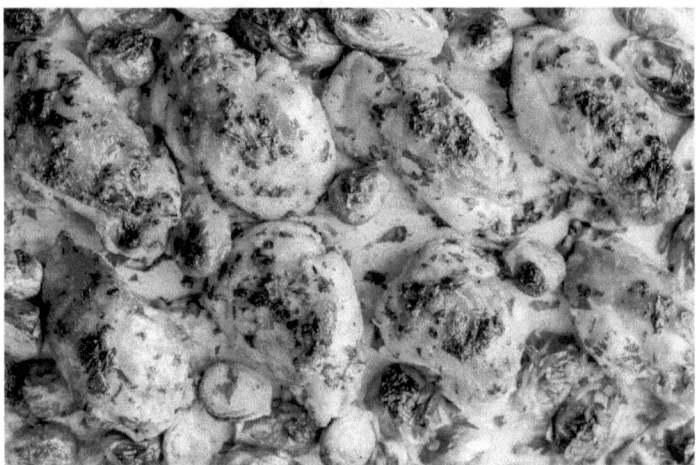

Ingredients:
- 4 chicken thighs (bone-in)
- 1 pound of brussel sprouts, trimmed and halved
- 3 tbsp olive oil
- 2 cloves garlic, minced
- 1 tsp dried thyme
- 1 tsp paprika
- Salt and crushed pepper to taste

Instructions:
- Preheat the oven to 400°F. Mix the olive oil, minced garlic, dried thyme, paprika, salt, and crushed pepper in a small bowl. Place the chicken thighs and Brussels sprouts in a large mixing bowl. Drizzle the olive oil mixture over the chicken and Brussels sprouts and toss to coat evenly.
- Arrange the chicken thighs and Brussels sprouts on a baking sheet with the chicken skin side up. Roast in the oven for 37-45 minutes until the chicken is cooked and the Brussels sprouts are tender and caramelized.
- Remove from the oven and let cool for 7-10 minutes before serving.

CHICKEN FRIED RICE

Calories: 309cal, Protein: 33g, Carbohydrate: 15g, Fat: 13g
Perp time: 10 minutes, Cook time: 25 minutes, Serving: 4

Ingredients:
- 2 chicken breasts without skin and bone diced
- 1 cup frozen peas and carrots
- 1 small onion, diced
- 3 cloves garlic, minced
- 2 eggs, lightly beaten
- 2 tbsp. of coconut oil
- 2 tbsp. of soy sauce
- 1 tsp. of sesame oil
- 1 cup cooked brown rice
- Salt and crushed pepper to taste
- Chopped green onions for garnish

Instructions:
- Heat one tbsp coconut oil in a non-stick skillet over medium-high heat. Add the diced chicken with salt and crushed pepper, and Cook until browned around for 5-7 minutes. Remove the chicken and set aside.
- Heat the leftover tbsp of coconut oil. Add the diced onion and cook for 3-4 minutes. Add garlic and cook for 30 seconds. Add the peas and carrots to the pan and cook until thawed about 5 minutes.
- Push the vegetables to one side of the pan and add the whisked eggs to the other side. Scramble the eggs until cooked through, then mix with the vegetables. Add the cooked brown rice to the pan and stir to combine.
- Add the cooked chicken with soy sauce and sesame oil and stir again to combine. Cook for 5 minutes or until the rice is heated through.
- Serve hot, garnished with chopped green onions.

"MY WEAKNESSES HAVE ALWAYS BEEN FOOD AND MEN- IN THAT ORDER."

DOLLY PARTON

PART III: AT-HOME WORKOUTS AND EXERCISE LIBRARY

AT-HOME WORKOUT ROUTINES

Get your body moving anywhere and everywhere! Use these at-home workout routines as a base to get your physical body moving regularly. You do not need any fitness equipment for these workout routines, just yourself, a mat (optional), a chair, and a positive mindset. Give these at-home workouts a try. Your body will thank you.

Consult with a physician before starting any new exercise program.

Beginner: 1-2 sets with 1–2-minute rest in between
Advanced: 2-3 Sets with 0:30-1 minute rest in between
Expert: 3-5 Sets with 0:30 rest on between

Circuit #1:
(Easiest)

20 High Knees
20 Bodyweight squats
12 Push-ups or modified push-ups
20 Reverse lunges (10 each leg)
:30 Forearm plank

Circuit #2:

20 Bodyweight squats
20 single-legged squats (10 on each side)
20 Walking lunges
20 Step up to balance
10 Tricep dips

Circuit #3:

12 Push-ups or modified push-ups
12 Tricep dips
20 Hip thrusters

:30 Forearm plank
20 Mountain climbers

Circuit #4:

20 Step up to balance
12 Inclined push-ups
20 Reverse lunges
12 Sit-ups
20 Hip thrusters

Circuit #5:
(Hardest)

20 High Knees
20 Mountain climbers
12 Tricep dips
20 Bodyweight squats
:30-1-minute forearm plank

Exercise Library:

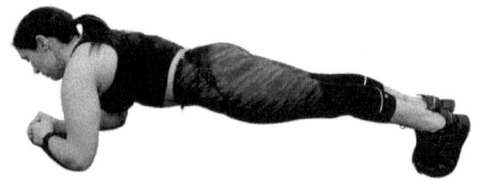

Forearm Plank

Muscles Activated: Rectus abdominis, Transversus abdominis, Internal oblique
Tips: Ensure your hips aren't dropping toward the
floor or hiking up toward the ceiling. Also, your shoulders are over your elbows.

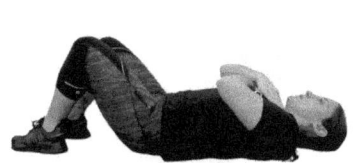 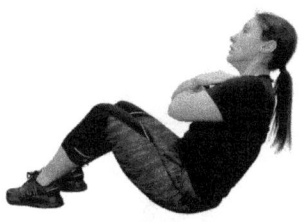

Sit-Ups

Muscles Activated: Rectus abdominis, Internal and external obliques, transverse abdominals, and hip flexors
Tips: Start in an upright sitting position on the ground, relax your shoulders, and keep your knees shoulder-width apart. Curl up in a C shape while inhaling and exhaling as you slowly rise, maintaining the C shape.

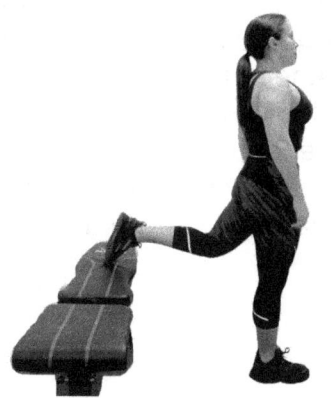 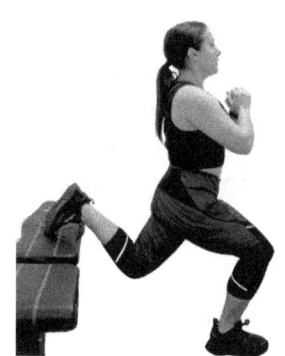

Split Squats

Muscles Activated: Hip flexors, hamstrings, quadriceps, and glutes.
Tips: Begin the movement by placing your knees at a 90-degree angle. Push up through the front foot. Keep your back straight and

core tight. Inhale when you go down and exhale when you push up.

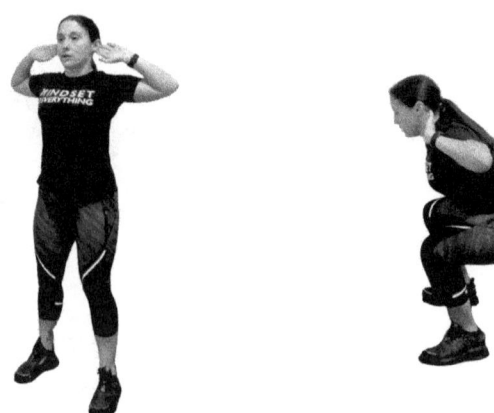

Bodyweight Squats

Muscles Activated: Lower Body (Glutes, Quads, Hamstrings)
Tips: Stand with your legs slightly wider than shoulder-width apart and your toes pointed outwards; keep your back straight and your eyes looking forward. Slowly bend your knees to a 90-degree angle and push your hips back so your thighs are parallel to the floor. Push your feet into the floor, squeeze your buttocks/glutes together and stand up tall. Modifications can include a sit-to-stand with a chair for beginners or jumping squats for a more advanced exercise.

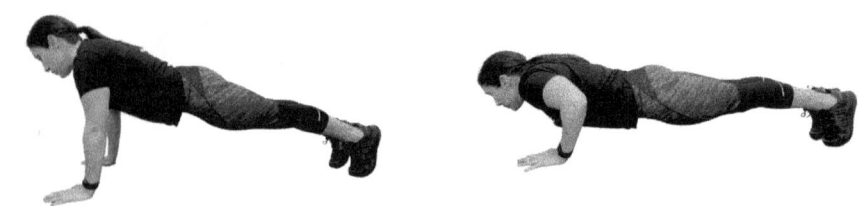

Push Ups

Muscles Activated: Pectoral muscles, shoulders, and triceps

Tips: Start in a high plank position, placing your hands slightly further than shoulder width. Lower your body until your chest nearly touches the ground. Push yourself back up and repeat. Modify as needed. Modifications of the push-up for beginners include knee push-ups, inclined push-ups, or wall push-ups.

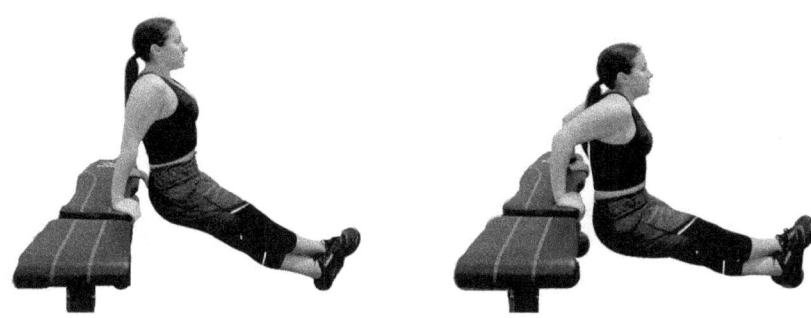

Tricep Dips

Muscles Activated: Triceps primarily, but also shoulders and pectoral muscles.

Tips: Face away from a chair or bench and grip the front edge. As you bend your arms and go down, your butt should be closely grazing the front of the chair or bench. Modifications include elevated tricep dips, weighted triceps dips and reverse plank tricep dips.

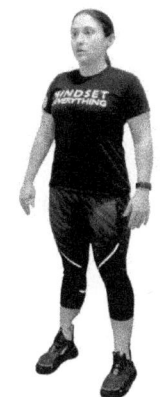
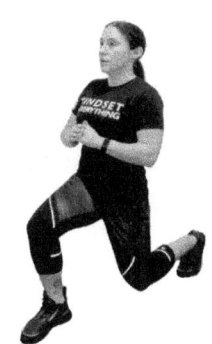

Reverse Lunges

Muscles Activated: Core, glutes and hamstrings.
Tips: Stand with your feet shoulder-width apart. Step backwards, landing on the ball of your foot and bending your knees to create two 90-degree angles. Push through your front heel to return to the standing position. Repeat on both legs.

High Knees

Muscles Activated: Quadriceps, hamstrings, calves, glutes, and hip flexors.
Tips: Stand with your feet forward, hip-width apart. Drive your knees toward your chest as high as possible while using your arms to gain momentum.
Keep your chest lifted and your core engaged, and land lightly on the balls of your feet. Modifications include a high knee march in place or a high knee march in a chair.

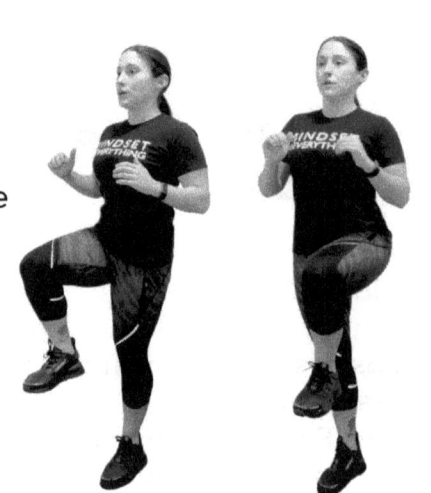

Mountain Climbers

Muscles Activated: Shoulders, hamstrings, core, triceps, and quadriceps.
Tips: Start in a push-up position. Keep your core engaged and drive your knees right to your chest.

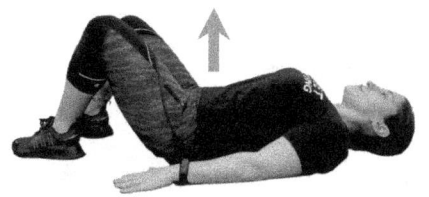 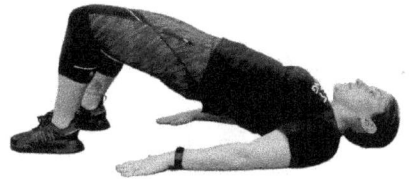

Hip Thrusters

Muscles Activated: Glutes and hip extensors—also your erector spinae (lower back), knee extensors, and quads.
Tips: Modify as needed. Start by lying flat on your back, knees bent, and your feet should be hip-distance apart. Squeeze into your buttocks and lift your hips, then lower them back down in a controlled manner.

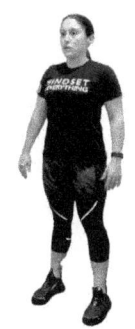 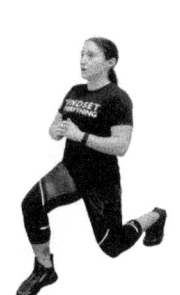 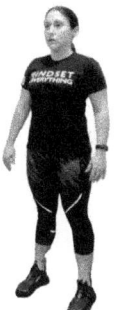 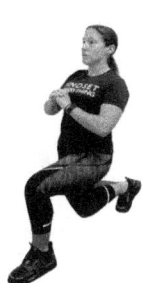

Walking Lunges

Muscles Activated: Gluteus maximus, hamstrings, quadriceps and gastrocnemius/soleus (calves)
Tips: Keep your shoulders back and chest upright and keep your core engaged. Step up far enough so your upper body can keep up straight and your hips are straight down.

Step-up to Balance

Muscles Activated: Quadriceps, hamstrings, and glutes.
Tips: Squeeze into your glutes and step onto the box or chair with one leg. Keep your shoulders back and your chest up. Make sure your feet and knees are facing forward.

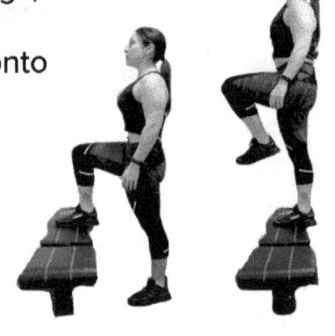

Single-Leg Bench Squats

Muscles Activated: Glutes, calves, quadriceps, hamstrings, and core.
Tips: Start by standing on your right foot. Keep your shoulders back and chest up with your core engaged. Squeeze your glutes as you stand back up. Repeat on both feet.

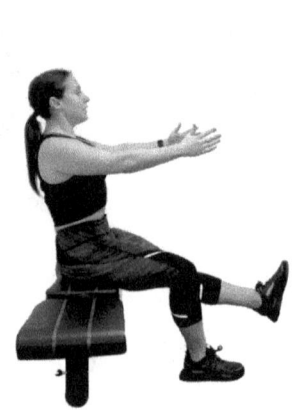 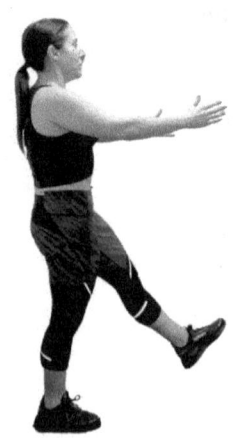

> "MY DAILY WORKOUT IS WHAT KEEPS ME FIT AND SANE."

GWYNETH PALTROW

MACRONUTRIENT CHEAT SHEET

MACRONUTRIENTS ARE NUTRIENTS THAT YOUR BODY USES IN THE LARGEST AMOUNT. THESE NUTRIENTS ARE WHERE YOUR BODY GETS ENERGY FROM.

A HEALTHY BALANCED DIET SHOULD NOT EXCLUDE OR SERIOUSLY RESTRICT ANY MACRONUTRIENT.

PROTEINS

CHICKEN
BEEF
PORK
FISH
TURKEY
SEAFOOD
EGGS
GREEK YOGURT
COTTAGE CHEESE
TOFU
WHEY
CASINE

FATS

CANOLA OIL
OLIVE OIL
AVOCADO OIL
COCONUT OIL
MAYONNAISE
BUTTER
NUT BUTTER
GHEE
FISH OIL
NUTS

CARBOHYDRATES

BREAD
RICE
OATMEAL
CEREAL
PASTA
CORN
NOODLES
QUINOA
TORTILLAS
FRUIT
VEGETABLES
POTATOES
TABLE SUGAR
BEANS
LENTILS

MACRONUTRIENT BREAKDOWN FOR WEIGHT LOSS

HIGH PROTEIN- 40-50%
LOW CARB- 10-30%
LOW FAT- 30-40%

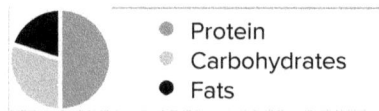

- Protein
- Carbohydrates
- Fats

REFERENCES

Bandini, Linda G et al. (2017) Changes in Food Selectivity in Children with Autism Spectrum Disorder. *Journal of Autism and Developmental Disorders* vol. 47,2, 439-446.

Bull FC, Al-Ansari SS, Biddle S, et al. World Health Organization. (2020) 2020 guidelines on physical activity and sedentary behaviour. *British Journal of Sports Medicine 2020;* 54:1451-1462.

Ellis, J.M., Zickgraf, H.F., Galloway, a.t. et al. (2018) A functional description of adult picky eating using latent profile analysis. *Int J Behav Nutr Phys Act* 15, 109.

McClaran, S. R. (2003). The effectiveness of personal training on changing attitudes towards physical activity. *Journal of Sports Medicine, pp. 2,* 10–14.

Painter SL, Ahmed R, Hill JO, et al. (2017) What Matters in Weight Loss? An In-Depth Analysis of Self-Monitoring. *J Med Internet Res.* 2017;19(5):e160.

Pearson ES. (2012). Goal setting as a health behaviour change strategy in overweight and obese adults: a systematic literature review examining intervention components. *Patient Educ Couns.* 87(1):32–42.

Popkin, B. M., D'Anci, K. E., & Rosenberg, I. H. (2010). Water, hydration, and health. *Nutrition Reviews, 68*(8), 439–458.

Rolls B. J. (2014). What is the role of portion control in weight management? *International journal of obesity*, p. *38 Suppl 1*, S1–S8.

Shain (2022). Yes, adults can be picky eaters. Here's how to stop. *Washington Post*

Stookey, J.D., Constant, F., Popkin, B.M. & Gardner, C.D. (2008). Drinking Water Is Associated With Weight Loss in Overweight Dieting Women Independent of Diet and Activity. *Obesity, pp. 16,* 2481–2488.

World Health Organization. (1999). Healthy living: what is a healthy lifestyle? *Copenhagen: WHO Regional Office for Europe.*

CLIENT TESTIMONIALS

Jess has completely transformed my fitness journey! With her expert guidance and personalized workouts, I have never felt stronger or more motivated to reach my fitness goals!

ADAM S., RICHMOND HILL, ON

Training with Jess has been extremely positive and beneficial for me. I always look forward to our sessions and she motivates me to drag myself to the gym in between. Jess is professional, punctual, knowledgeable, encouraging and realistic when helping me to set goals. She "gets it" and pushes me just the right amount. I would highly recommend Jess as a trainer for people of all ages and with varying needs.

ANDREA B., TORONTO, ON.

My time working with Jess has not only been exhilarating, but it has also been an incredible learning experience. It's very easy to feel comfortable around her, and I always feel supported and motivated during every workout. Jess makes me feel like I can accomplish so much more than I ever knew I could. It's a great feeling to connect with somebody who understands where you are coming from. I look forward to all of my sessions, and that's all because of Jess and her motivational and encouraging attitude.

BRITNEY K., THORNHILL, ON.

We have been working out with Jess since 2019. She is always super positive and energetic! Even if you aren't feeling your best, she will motivate and encourage you to keep trying. Her favourite expression is, "You've got this!" She listens well to what your goals are, takes into account your stage of life, and puts an action plan together. We highly recommend Jess as a personal trainer and can attest that she lives by her motto, "Mindset is Everything!" We look forward to working with her for many more years to come.

CAROL AND CARL, VAUGHAN, ON.

Since I started training with Jess at the beginning of 2022, I have lost almost 72 pounds by following her approach to weight loss and adopting a healthy lifestyle. Jess is like no other trainer I have ever used before and I recommend her to anyone wanting to lose weight, get healthy and be their best self. She has taught, motivated, and inspired me to keep going and only become happier, healthier and stronger one step at a time.

JACOB S., TORONTO, ON.

I have always lived a healthy lifestyle by eating well and exercising regularly. I take dance classes and practice yoga for about 10 hours a week. However, I never considered myself a "gym person". In 2019, I reached out to Jess with the singular goal of toning my arms in preparation for our studio's 30th-anniversary dance showcase. Although the show was sadly cancelled due to the COVID lockdown, four years later, I'm still training with Jess on a weekly basis. The benefits I've received from interval training with Jess have been immense. Coming out of a pandemic, I feel more toned, balanced, and physically and mentally stronger than ever before. Jess is an attentive listener, an engaging trainer, and a wonderful motivator. She always customizes the program to accommodate my needs and how my body feels each week. She makes the sessions fun and has effectively converted a "gym phobic" to a high-intensity training enthusiast. Thank you, Jess!

NASHEEN L., TORONTO, ON.

ACKNOWLEDGMENTS

I want to thank my incredibly supportive parents, Sheila and Steve, for their endless love and support. From supporting every crazy idea I have ever had to inspire me to be a better person every day, I could not have done all this without you both by my side cheering me on.

I also want to thank my brother, my sister-in-law, my nephews, and everyone else who has supported me along this journey, including my extended family and friends. This book is for all of you.

Lastly, I want to thank and acknowledge all the people who have body-shamed me, bullied me, told me no, or tried to knock me down; thank you. Each and every experience has made me stronger, and I have learned to love myself and my body even more, so thank you all.

This is all God's plan, and I can't wait to see what comes next!

STAY POSITIVE AND STAY STRONG!

#FIVEFOOTSTRONG

ABOUT THE AUTHOR

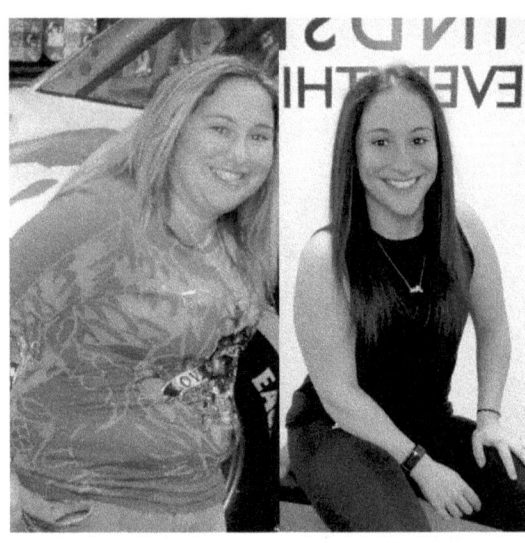

Jessica Gerlock is a certified personal trainer from Vaughan, Ontario. In 2014, she lost over 100 pounds at 22 years old after being considered overweight and clinically obese for most of her childhood and adolescence. Jessica now motivates and inspires others daily with her healthy lifestyle approach and positive attitude. She is certified through the National Academy of Sports Medicine, holding current specializations as a Weight Loss Specialist, Performance Enhancement Specialist, Corrective Exercise Specialist and Youth Exercise Specialist.

Jessica is the head trainer of Mindset Fitness and Wellness, a business which provides in-home and virtual personal training services to men and women of all ages. She has helped countless people achieve their fitness and weight loss goals. Jessica has also written fitness blogs for *PopSugar*, *Dove*'s BeReal Campaign, *#SickNotWeak*, *Huffington Post* and jessicagerlock.com. Jessica has appeared on multiple podcasts, radio and TV shows, sharing her weight loss journey and personal struggles with dealing with mental health. For more information on Jessica and her journey, please visit www.JessicaGerlock.com.

www.ingramcontent.com/pod-product-compliance
Lightning Source LLC
Chambersburg PA
CBHW060032040426
42333CB00042B/2316